THOMAS MCKEOWN

The Origins of
HUMAN
DISEASE

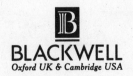

BLACKWELL
Oxford UK & Cambridge USA

Copyright © Thomas McKeown, 1988

First published 1988
First published in paperback 1991
Reprinted 1993, 1994, 1995

Blackwell Publishers Ltd.
108 Cowley Road, Oxford OX4 1JF, UK

Blackwell Publishers Inc.
238 Main Street
Cambridge, Massachusetts 02142, USA

British Library Cataloguing in Publication Data
A CIP catalogue record for this book is available from the British Library.

Library of Congress Cataloging in Publication Data
A CIP catalogue record for this book is available from the Library of Congress.
ISBN 0-631-17938-0

Typeset in 10 on 12 pt Baskerville
by Downdell Ltd, Abingdon, Oxon.
Printed and bound in Great Britain
by Hartnolls Limited, Bodmin, Cornwall

This book is printed on acid-free paper

Contents

Preface

In this book I have tried to bring together two subjects which are generally considered separately, but which seem to me to be properly regarded as related parts of a larger whole. One subject, historical demography, is concerned with the study of the size of human populations; the other, a relatively neglected area of medical history, deals with the origins of disease and assesses the part played by medical and other influences in bringing about past changes in health.

When writing about these matters, or discussing them in lectures or seminars, I have found myself in contact with two essentially different groups of people. The demographic theme has been of interest chiefly to demographers and economic historians, for whom the relation between population growth and economic and industrial development is a major issue. They have been particularly concerned with the early phase of industrialization in the eighteenth and nineteenth centuries, and with the questions of whether improved economic conditions led to expansion of population, or whether the growth of population which assisted industrial-ization was due to to some other cause essentially independent of it. These interests have brought historians to the study of fertility and mortality, and to what should be common ground with the medical historian, assessment of reasons for changes in health in the past.

Remarkably, medical historians have had little to say about the history of human health, mainly, I believe, because they thought the explanation was self-evident. Since the seventeenth century medical thinking has been dominated by the concept of the body as a machine, whose protection from disease and its effects depends primarily on internal intervention. The modern improvement of health was assumed to be due to advances in medical knowledge applied through clinical preventive and therapeutic procedures, and the possibility that health was being transformed by profound changes in conditions of life was not seriously considered. Hence, histories of medicine, like histories of art, have two main themes, the great men and the great movements: Leonardo and the High Renaissance; Pasteur and the rise of bacteriology. Historians have written about the lives and works of Hippocrates, Galen, Paracelsus and Osler, but they have not inquired whether the treatments of the great physicians were of benefit to their patients. They have been concerned with the description of significant events in medical history, rather than with examination of the part that medicine and other influences have played in relation to human health. Even Sigerist, the distinguished historian who recognized the need for enlargement of medical historical interests, did not make a clear distinction between that doctors were doing and what they were achieving.

If you open a textbook, any textbook, of medical history and try to find what health conditions were like in rural France in the eighteenth century, or what disease meant to the family of an artisan in the same period, you will as a rule not find any information. We know much about the great medical discoveries but very little on whether they were applied, or to whom they were applied.

This extract from Sigerist's essay on 'The Social History of Medicine' suggests that in spite of his broad concept of medical history, he did not recognize that the great discoveries were not necessarily, or indeed usually, followed by any immediate benefits to the sick. It is important to know that three and a half centuries after the discovery of the circulation of the blood, the risk of a heart attack is much greater (because of smoking), and the risk of death from an attack little less, than it was in Harvey's day.

The second group of people with whom I have been in contact, particularly since the publication of my book on the role of medicine,[1] is comprised mainly of physicians, although latterly it has also included sociologists, economists and others concerned with health policies. For them the interest has been not so much in historical interpretation as in the significance of the conclusions for contemporary medicine. For many physicians the finding that medical intervention had little effect on mortality before the twentieth century has been no more than an academic endorsement of their own experience. But others have found it difficult to accept that treatment of disease was less effective than other influences, and some regard discussion of these matters as an attack on clinical medicine. It was not so intended, and indeed my own conclusion is that although the nature of the contribution of medicine is somewhat different from what it was formerly considered to be, it is no less important. Paradoxically, the healthier we are the longer we live, and the longer we live the more likely we are to require the benefit from medical care. In this book I have sought to find more neutral ground and, to change the metaphor, to cover a larger canvas. I

[1] McKeown T. *The Role of Medicine*. Oxford, Basil Blackwell, 1979.

have tried to classify diseases according to their origins and to consider the significance of the conclusions for the future control of disease.

As life must be possible before it can be pleasant ('a pair of boots is of more value than all the plays of Shakespeare'[2]), human health and its relation to conditions of life and population growth are among the great themes of history. Why did early man, although apparently well adapted to his environment, have high death rates and a short expectation of life? Why did the change from hunting and gathering to agriculture lead to the predominance of infectious diseases as causes of sickness and death? Where, among the nutritional, environmental, behavioural and medical advances of the last three centuries, are we to find the explanation for the modern improvement in health? And are the most serious threats to health in the future likely to come from the infections or from non-communicable diseases, a question brought sharply to public attention by the appearance of AIDS? These are some of the questions to be considered, and we are more likely to find the answers if they are examined together.

I am indebted to my friends and former colleagues Professor E. G. Knox and Professor J. M. Bishop for valuable suggestions. Professor Knox has read the whole of the text and Professor Bishop chapters 5 and 8 which deal with subjects on which he has had extensive experience. My special thanks are owed to Mrs Christine Harlow who has typed the book from an unsightly script and worked patiently on its revision.

[2] A remark attributed to the Russian critic Pisarev by Isaiah Berlin. In: *Against the Current*. London, The Hogarth Press, 1979.

Introduction

The present time is, arguably, the first when a comprehensive attempt to interpret the relation between conditions of life, health and population growth can profitably be made. Before the nineteenth century ideas concerning disease origins were, to say the least, confused. Infectious diseases were attributed to miasmas, non-communicable diseases were a mystery, and many people denied a relation between living conditions and health. For although it has long been evident that people who are sick are often poor, it has not always been recognized that many of them are sick because they are poor. It was thought that the sick poor were, in some ill-defined way, intrinsically inferior, and that an improvement in their circumstances would have little effect on their health and perhaps only a temporary effect on their poverty. In preferring five pounds he would be happy to spend to ten pounds he would be unhappy to save, Mr. Doolittle in Shaw's *Pygmalion* would have been regarded as typical of people for whom little could be done in respect of health or wealth by public action.

The nineteenth century removed misunderstandings about the nature of infectious diseases; but for non-communicable diseases such as cancer, diabetes and heart disease, the same notions persisted until the second half of the twentieth century, and it is only in the last few decades that evidence of their environmental and behavioural origins has accumulated to the point where it can no longer be seriously disputed. The health scene can now be likened to a large and complex jig-saw puzzle, of which at last enough pieces are visible to enable them to be fitted into a recognizable whole. Many sources have contributed to the picture, but the following are among the key discoveries.

1 Recognition that human genetic constitution is much the same today as it was 100,000 years ago, before the advent of any pastoral, agricultural or industrial activity. We now face vastly changed conditions of life with the genetic equipment of hunter gatherers.

2 The finding that in technological advanced countries the modern transformation of health, and the associated increase of population, began more than a century before effective medical intervention was possible, and must be attributed largely to advances in the standard of living.

3 The discovery by medical science of the nature of infectious diseases and the possibility of their prevention by increasing resistance and reducing exposure.

4 Recognition in the last few decades that most classes of non-communicable diseases also have environmental origins and are potentially preventable by changes in living conditions and behaviour.

The health of man, as of other living things, is determined by both positive and negative requirements, by the satisfaction of basic needs and by avoidance of serious hazards. There are four basic needs – food, oxygen, warmth (or, more accurately, avoidance of excessive heat loss) and water – perceptively identified by the ancients as the four elements – earth, air, fire and water. In relation to health it is significant that the length of time for which people can survive without the essentials is inversely related to their availability: oxygen for minutes; heat for hours; water for days; and food for weeks.

Human life is impossible unless oxygen is immediately available, and over most of the earth's surface it is virtually unlimited. Warmth and water are almost equally necessary for immediate use, and it is only to a limited extent that man needs to increase the amounts of these essentials. When he does so it is mainly for other purposes, as in the damming of rivers to obtain power or food, or because he has exposed himself to deficiencies by visiting or living in very cold or dry climates. Oxygen, warmth and water are, so to speak, the 'given' requirements for health, and we cannot survive where they are seriously deficient. We can live in the foothills of high mountains but not at their peaks, in sub-arctic tundra but not near the poles, at the periphery of large deserts but not at the centre. Lack of oxygen, shelter or water is only an infrequent cause of sickness or death, and man's restless wandering to remote parts of the earth has not been in search for these essentials. It is the need for them that will curb his intrusion in outer space.

The position in respect of the fourth basic need is quite different, in that the supply is strictly limited. Man needs proteins which can be obtained only by consumption of plants and other animals; the size of animal populations is determined ultimately by the amount of plant food; and plants, which can synthesize the amino acids that animals require, depend in turn on ingredients available in a narrow band which extends only a few inches below the earth's surface. In the strictest sense it is true to say that life requires destruction of the living and consumption of the ashes of the dead, a bitter truth beautifully expressed in one of the most striking passages in modern verse:

> You whom I gladly walk with, touch,
> Or wait for as one certain of good,
> We know it; we know that love
> Needs more than the admiring excitement of union;
> More than the abrupt self-confident farewell,
> The heel on the finishing blade of grass,
> The self-confidence of the falling root.
> Needs death, death of the grain, our death,
> Death of the old gang; would leave them
> In sullen valley where is made no friend,
> The old gang to be forgotten in the spring
> The hard bitch and the riding-master,
> Stiff underground; deep in clear lake
> The lolling bridegroom, beautiful, there.[1]

In fact man's food resources are far below the level determined by the basic restraints. A considerable amount of plant protein in grass and leaves is not available for human consumption unless converted to another form, as in the milk of cows or goats. Even today, although marginal areas are increasingly cultivated, much of the land suitable for agriculture is either not used or produces below its capacity. Hence, although productivity can be increased, there are strict limits to the size of population that can be fed. Unlike the other essentials, therefore, food is not 'given'; it has to be gathered, hunted, cultivated, preserved and at times competed for. It is the critical determinant of health and population growth, and a pivotal question is whether, as Malthus believed, the limits it imposes are commonly reached: 'The tendency of all animated life is to increase beyond the nourishment prepared for it.'

But health is also prejudiced by serious hazards, which may arise naturally or may be man-made. For most living things the natural hazards are from predators and parasites; but man is fortunate in having no natural predators, that is other animals which kill in order to consume human flesh. There are, of course, the analogous phenomena of war and cannibalism: man is almost unique in killing his own kind; but the killing is not mainly to satisfy hunger, and cannibalism has always been uncommon. In any case it is man-made, so that among natural hazards the chief threat to health has been, and remains, from parasites.

[1] Auden, W. H. *Poems*. London, Faber & Faber Ltd., 1934: 66.

In this context parasites are taken to include all organisms, both micro-scopic and macroscopic, which feed on the living host and only inadvertently cause death. It is clearly to the advantage of the parasite to have a healthy and well-nourished host, and where the two have been in close contact for a considerable time the resulting relationship is generally benign, and sometimes mutually beneficial. Through natural selection the hosts acquire resistance to organisms which cause disease, by their ability to produce an immune response and by the more general type of intrinsic resistance which makes an individual immune to a particular organism. It is this last type of immunity which explains why shigella dysentery is confined to primates and Johne's disease to ruminants, why most children exposed to poliomyelitis virus do not suffer from the disease, and why tuberculosis is a natural infection of man, cattle, pigs and fowls but is relatively uncommon in sheep, goats, horses and dogs. By natural selection micro-organisms also adapt, and the relationship can be said to be in balance in the sense that there are reciprocal changes in organism and host. There are, however, some well-defined circumstances in which serious disease may occur.

1 When organisms are encountered for the first time or after an interval of several generations, as in explosive infections from plague, typhus and influenza. In the case of viruses Andrewes noted that when an infection is introduced to a strange host one of three things may occur: the virus may fail to multiply and this, probably the commonest outcome, passes unnoticed; the virus may multiply and kill the host without being transmitted to another, in which case the infection ends at this point; after a period of adaptation, accompanied initially by sickness and even death of some hosts and parasites, the viruses and their hosts may settle in a relation of mutual tolerance not normally associated with disease. The serious disease which arises from fresh contact with parasites is usually short-lived.[2]

2 Where the survival of the organism is promoted by the sickness of the host: the common cold is spread by sneezing, cholera by diarrhoea, respiratory tuberculosis by coughing and rabies by the biting of dogs. While such examples are to be found among organisms that cause sickness and death, they are very uncommon in micro-organisms as a whole.

3 Where the relationship between host and parasite is seriously disturbed. This is usually attributed to ecological imbalance or

[2] Andrewes, C. *Viruses and Evolution.* University of Birmingham, The Huxley Lecture, 1965–66.

stress; but these terms do not specify the nature of the disturbance, and it is more precise to say that the common, although perhaps not the only causes, are crowding and lack of food. Moreover, it is possible – to claim no more – that the two are related, that the stress from crowding results largely from the threat or reality of food deficiency.

With due regard for such exceptions, the general conclusion that has been drawn is that when hosts and parasites evolve together for a considerable time, the hosts develop efficient mechanisms of resistance and the infections are of low virulence.[3] The trend is from virulence to commensalism, and according to this view parasites do not play a large part in limiting population growth by causing disease. However, it should be said that this conclusion is accepted by some people only with reservations. It has been argued on theoretical grounds that co-evolution does not preclude stable long term associations between virulent parasites and their hosts,[4, 5] and they are said to have occurred in (for example) the persistence of highly virulent strains of smallpox virus in India, and the apparently stable virulent virus/host association in rabbits infected by myxomatosis.[6] However, such relationships are also exceptional, and most long-term parasite/host associations are relatively benign unless disturbed by major changes in conditions of life.

To complete this introductory appraisal of influences on human health it is necessary to recognize that many serious hazards, and today probably most, are man-made. In prehistoric times they resulted largely from hunting and gathering, homicide in various forms, and penetration into inhospitable parts of the world, usually in search for food. But greater risks have come from the profound changes associated with the development of agriculture and industrialization. Moreover, these changes have occurred in what is, on an evolutionary timescale, a very short period, so that we are genetically ill-equipped for the ways of life that we have made for ourselves. A school child eating potato crisps while watching television, a driver steering a bus or taxi through a congested city, an adolescent smoking in front of a computer, are far removed from the conditions for which their

[3] Allison, A. C. 'Co-evolution between hosts and infectious disease agents and its effects on virulence.' In: Anderson, R. M. and May, R. M. (eds) *Population Biology of Infectious Diseases*. Berlin, Springer-Verlag, 1982: 245.

[4] Anderson, R. M. and May, R. M. 'Co-evolution of hosts and parasites.' *Parasitology*, 1982.

[5] Anderson, R. M. and May, R. M. 'Population biology of infectious diseases: Part II' *Nature*, 1979, **280**: 455–61.

[6] Levin, B. R. 'Evolution of parasites and hosts: group report.' In: Anderson, R. M. and May, R. M. (eds) *Population Biology of Infectious Diseases*. Berlin, Springer-Verlag, 1982: 219.

genes have prepared them. One of the paradoxes to be explained is why health has improved in spite of such adverse influences.

In this introduction I have touched briefly on several themes which will be developed in later chapters. Part I is concerned with the relation between conditions of life and health and population growth in the three major periods into which human existence naturally falls. For hunter-gatherers (chapter 1), the most important question which arises is whether numbers were in general maintained below the level that the food resources of the environment could support. If we believe that they were, we must account in other ways for the shortness of life and slow rate of population growth; if we believe they were not, we are led to Malthus' view that both were determined directly or indirectly by food deficiency. We must also come to a conclusion about early man's experience of both infectious and non-communicable diseases.

In the agricultural period (chapter 2) there are several important and related questions. Did expansion of populations precede or follow developments in agriculture? Why did the change in way of life lead to the predominance of infectious diseases as causes of sickness and death? What was the source of the human infections which were rare or absent in hunter-gatherers?

In the industrial period (chapter 3) we must consider some questions about which there is still disagreement. Was the modern rise of population due mainly to an increase of the birth rate or to a decrease of the death rate? Why did mortality from infectious diseases decline in the period when exposure to them initially increased? What parts have medicine and other influences played in bringing about the transformation of health in the past two centuries? Is the predominance of non-communicable diseases in developed countries attributable essentially to genetic susceptibility or to changes in conditions of life?

To provide insight into the feasibility and means of disease control we require a classification of diseases, not on the usual physiological or pathological lines, but according to disease origins. The clearest distinction that can be made is between diseases determined irreversibly at fertilization and those – the large majority – not so determined and manifested only in an appropriate environment. Although genetic constitution is important in relation to the latter, such diseases are potentially preventable by control of the environmental component. The diseases determined at fertilization cannot be prevented in this way, but must be dealt with by other means – contraception, abortion, treatment, modification of genes or chromosomes – measures which are based on knowledge of disease mechanisms. As a basis for a strategy of preventive and therapeutic measures, however, and having regard for the predominant influences on human health at different periods of existence, a three-fold classification (as in Part II) is more instructive, taking together all diseases determined before birth (prenatal diseases) – whether at fertilization or later in the uterus – and dividing conditions determined after birth according to whether they are due to deficiencies and hazards (diseases of poverty) or to maladaptation and hazards (diseases of affluence).

The prenatal diseases (chapter 4) comprise both abnormalities determined at fertilization and those not so determined which are due to influences within the uterus. It is unlikely that they include any of the so-called 'common diseases'. The prenatal diseases can be thought of as the price to be paid for the advantages which accrue from the intricate exchange of genes at fertilization or from the protection afforded by a prolonged period of intra-uterine life.

The diseases due to deficiencies and hazards (chapter 5) are essentially the diseases of poverty. However, an important distinction must be made between their modes of operation before and after the first agricultural revolution. The causes of ill-health in the hunter-gatherer period were distinguished from those that followed chiefly by a different experience of infectious disease. As a result of the social and economic advances of the last three centuries diseases due to deficiencies and natural hazards are no longer the principal cause of sickness and death in industrialized countries, but in large parts of the world the picture remains essentially unchanged.

Conditions of life during the last few thousand years, and (in developed countries) particularly in the last few hundred, have changed profoundly from those under which man evolved. In these short intervals there has not been time for major genetic adaptation. Chapter 6 examines the grounds for believing that most non-communicable diseases are due to changes in living conditions and behaviour associated with industrialization.

Part III is concerned with the significance of the analysis of disease origins for disease control. The relatively intractable character of most prenatal abnormalities (discussed in chapter 7) is evident from the fact that in developed countries they have not responded to the advances in conditions of life which have been so successful with postnatal diseases. With some important exceptions (due to low birth weight, iodine deficiency, radiation and the like) prenatal diseases are unlikely to be prevented by control of environmental and behavioural influences, and must be tackled by other means which depend on knowledge of their mechanisms. This indeed is the field which uniquely requires the traditional laboratory and clinical approaches, and the more successful preventive measures are in dealing with postnatal conditions, the more important the residual prenatal problems will be seen to be.

For much of the world the diseases of poverty (chapter 8) are still predominant. The measures required for their prevention are well known – the provision of sufficient and safe food, clean water, sanitation, immunization and limitation of numbers. The deficiencies are rooted in poverty, and the action needed is largely outside the control of health departments. Moreover, the diseases of poverty are by no means restricted to the developing world, and in the wealthiest countries there are sections of the population which are inadequately, as distinct from unwisely, fed.

Under this same heading we must also consider diseases of the tropics, both infectious and non-communicable, which were absent or uncommon in temperate climates. Conceptually they belong to the diseases of poverty, in the sense that they are due to deficiencies and hazards and could be prevented if resources were unlimited, in the extreme case by removal of populations from hazardous areas. In principle, people could avoid those parts of the world where there are high risks from parasites, just as they avoid those areas where there are high risks from cold. In practice, however, resources are severely limited, and as the tropical diseases frequently do not respond to simple improvements in conditions of life, the solution must come from new knowledge obtained from laboratory, clinical, epidemiological and socio-economic research.

The last chapter (9) is concerned with some of the major health problems now facing developed countries. It is only in the last few decades that it has begun to be recognized that the non-communicable diseases are not to be regarded as a hard core of genetically determined conditions, previously obscured by the shortness of life and the predominance of the infections. Most are due to environmental and behavioural changes associated with industrialization, and the challenge to society is to identify and reverse the influences that are responsible. Some of them are already known, and delay in advance is due more to personal behaviour and social policies than to lack of knowledge.

Finally I should consider briefly the possible criticism that discussion of these matters is not scientific because many of the conclusions are not capable of disproof. The same might be said of evolution through natural selection, and if the Almighty were to present us with a new species from outer space, apparently unrelated to all known antecedents, we would not necessarily reject the theory of evolution as an interpretation of human origins on earth. What we are seeking is an interpretation of a series of interrelated events, not a universal law which would be invalidated by a single exception. Very general theories are not isolated conjectures which can be shown to be wrong but not to be right; they are frameworks of thought, complex conceptual schemes for assembling and interpreting data. They are tested for usefulness and fertility in many ways, of which no single one is conclusive, and they are of value even if all that can be said in retrospect is that, like the curate's egg, they are good in parts.

But although I do not think that the test of falsifiability is relevant to most of the ideas outlined in this book, I see the force of the advice that 'whenever we propose a solution to a problem, we ought to try as hard as we can to overthrow our solution, rather than defend it.'[7] I shall therefore refer briefly to some points on which the interpretation of the relation between conditions of life and health and population growth may be questioned, either because it is unsupported by evidence or because it seems to be inconsistent with it.

One of the most important points which arises in the history of human health is whether population growth was effectively restrained in the hunter-gatherer period by control of fertility and postnatal killing. Whether early man was healthy, the causes of ill health, and the reasons for the slow rate of population growth before 8,000 BC, all turn on the answer to this question. It has to be said that conclusive data are not available, and the answer rests on indirect evidence which some will interpret differently.

For demographers one of the most persistent questions is whether the modern rise of population was due mainly to an increase in fertility or a reduction of mortality. In a sense this seems to me to be a secondary issue, since if we exclude medical measures and fortuitous change in the character of infectious diseases as important reasons for the decline of mortality in the last three centuries, we are led to the conclusion that improvement in economic and social conditions was the reason for the change in the birth rate or the death rate. But I know that in attaching much greater importance to the decline of mortality I appear to be ignoring the extensive work on parish registers which has suggested that an increase of the birth rate was the predominant influence before the mid-nineteenth century. I should therefore explain that I do not think there is any treatment of the deficient material from the registers that would make it reliable, and I have preferred to base conclusions on later and, in general, more trustworthy evidence.

Some will undoubtedly question the conclusions I have drawn concerning the predominant role of nutrition: that the slow growth of the human population before the eighteenth century was due mainly to high mortality caused by lack of food; that the rapid increase from that time resulted largely from improved nutrition; and that the influence of food on health and population growth in the historical period was determined essentially by the relation between nutritional state and response to infectious disease. Initially I came to these conclusions through rejection of other explanations for the modern increase in population size, on the principle enunciated by Sherlock Holmes: *When we have eliminated the impossible, whatever remains,*

[7] Popper, K. R. *The Logic of Scientific Discovery*. London, Hutchinson, 1959: 16.

however improbable, must be the truth. I had concluded that: (a) personal medical measures (immunization and therapy) had an insignificant effect on mortality before the twentieth century; (b) variations in the character of some infectious diseases is an inadequate general explanation for the major changes in man's experience of them; (c) the expansion and aggregation of populations which followed industrialization initially increased exposure to the infections; and (d) the ways in which it is suggested that fertility was restricted before the nineteenth century were relatively ineffective. However, I now believe that the conclusions concerning nutrition also rest on positive grounds, on a reading of the determinants of health and of the major influences which have modified it in the past, and on extensive experience of infectious diseases in relation to nutrition in the Third World.

In general it will be seen that I am doubtful about the reliability of much historical evidence related to health, unless it has been screened critically through present-day experience. Assertions are often made about the past which appear to be quite inconsistent with what we now know; for example: that abortion was an effective population control procedure before anaesthesia and antisepsis were known; that the nutrition of children did not greatly influence their response to infection;[8, 9] that some eighteenth-century hospitals achieved much better results than modern hospitals;[10] that children were fed, and the fertility of mothers effectively suppressed, by breast feeding for periods of two years or more; that inoculation against smallpox in the eighteenth century had an effect on mortality far greater than any modern immunization procedure;[11] that infectious diseases in earlier centuries can be diagnosed from the seasonal distribution of deaths; that Kung Bushmen could walk 34 miles in 5 hours on sand, a rate only a little lower than the Olympic record for about a fifth of the distance (on hard ground).[12] This list, which could easily be lengthened, is perhaps sufficient to show that some historical evidence related to health is questionable, and should not be accepted if inconsistent with present-day knowledge.

Fortunately, there is a good deal of contemporary experience which

[8] Watkins, S. C. and Van de Walle, E. 'Nutrition, mortality and population size: Malthus' court of last resort.' In: Rotberg, R. I. and Rabb, T. K. (eds) *Hunger and History.* Cambridge, Cambridge University Press, 1983: 21.

[9] Livi-Bacci, M. 'The nutrition-mortality link in past times.' In: Rotberg, R. I. and Rabb, T. K. (eds) *Hunger and History.* Cambridge, Cambridge University Press, 1983: 100.

[10] Sigsworth, E. 'A provincial hospital in the eighteenth and early nineteenth centuries.' *Yorkshire Faculty Journal,* 1966, **XVI**: 24.

[11] Razzell, P. E. 'Population change in eighteenth century England: a reinterpretation.' *Economic History Review,* 1965, **XVIII**: 312.

[12] Barnes, F. 'The biology of pre-neolithic man.' In: Boyden, S. W. (ed.) *The Impact of Civilization on the Biology of Man.* Toronto, University of Toronto Press, 1970: 11.

throws light on health in the past. In the world today there are examples of almost all the forms of social organization that have ever existed: the hunter-gatherers of prehistoric times; the nomadic pastoralists and primitive agriculturalists; the unhygienic large cities characteristic of early industrial development; and the complex modern societies of the developed world.[14] There is also considerable experience of other animals, including primates, in their natural habitats. Some of this evidence is transient and will soon be lost if it is not recorded. The planes which descend on to primitive airstrips in remote parts of Asia, Africa and Latin America, carry people who bring their infections and ways of life; and although the tourists are immunized, well fed, and coached to avoid the hazards of the primitive life, the residents are ill-equipped to meet the threats from the tourists. The few surviving hunter-gatherers already show signs of contact with other people, and the disease patterns of pastoralists and primitive agriculturalists are changing rapidly under the influence of the western life style. There will soon be few people in the world who live under the conditions that have prevailed for almost the whole of man's existence. If this is the first time that the problems of human health can be seen in an international and historical perspective, it may also be the last.

To complete this introduction I must explain briefly the reasons for limiting the subject matter of this book to physical disease. There would appear to be good reasons for considering also the origins of mental illness. The importance of increased understanding of psychiatric problems can hardly be exaggerated. In developed countries during the last few centuries there has been no improvement in mental health comparable to that in physical health; nor is knowledge so far advanced, and it could not be said of the one, as of the other, that the full application of what is known would greatly reduce the size of the problem. Moreover it is evident that the size and character of mental health problems, like those of physical health, are determined largely by the environment and behaviour: 'if the conditions of life of an animal deviate from those which prevailed in the environment in which the species evolved, the likelihood is that the animal will be less well suited to the new conditions than to those to which it has become genetically adapted through natural selection and consequently some signs of maladjustment may be anticipated'[13] The frequency of some problems has undoubtedly increased in developed countries: for example, longer expectation of life has resulted in survival to late ages where certain psychiatric illnesses are more common; it has also increased the number of

[13] Boyden, S. V. 'Evolution and Health.' *Ecologist*, 1973: 3, 304–09.

[14] Fenner, F. 'The effects of changing social organization on the infectious diseases of man.' In: Boyden, S. W. (ed.) *The Impact of Civilization on the Biology of Man.* Toronto, University of Toronto Press, 1970: 48–68.

mentally disabled and handicapped people, many of whom would formerly have died early in life. Directly or indirectly, changes associated with industrialization and affluence have created psychiatric problems from drug abuse, suicide, promiscuity and the like. Even developing countries have not escaped, and the consequences of changing conditions of life on mental health are to be seen in the alienation of the unfortunate people displaced from their rural homelands to slums at the periphery of large cities.

But although the problems of physical and mental health have a good deal in common, there are important differences. In the case of physical illness, the nature of the predominant health problems has been determined essentially by the prevailing conditions of life, and a fairly clear distinction can be made between diseases caused by poverty – chiefly the infections – and non-communicable diseases which have resulted from industrialization and affluence. In the case of mental illness, although elimination of poverty and restraints on affluence would undoubtedly have beneficial effects, there is not the same clear cut relation between these influences and specific diseases. It is for this reason that it has seemed advisable to limit the analysis of disease origins and control to physical disease.

PART I

Disease History

1

Hunting and Gathering

Seed-bag and Urn

Until recently many of our ideas about living things were based on observations of animals domesticated or maintained in the artificial environments of laboratories and zoos. In the last few years, however, television has provided an impressive account of the conditions of life and behaviour of plants and animals in their natural habitats. The record is now much more extensive than that which was available to Darwin in his years with the Beagle, for it includes not only observations made in all parts of the world, but microscopic and other evidence from remote and inaccessible places – underwater, after dark and in deserts and polar regions. Indeed if evolution by natural selection were not already known, it is conceivable that some bright adolescent, equipped with Malthus' essay and a television set, would soon discover it.

In these intimate pictures animals are seen to be engaged chiefly in two occupations, acquiring or consuming food and reproducing, although attention has also to be given to protecting themselves and their offspring from predators engaged in the same pursuits. Nature is indeed red in tooth and claw, and only those equipped to meet the triple threats of predator, parasite and food shortage can survive and reproduce. Under natural conditions, living things appear to be at the mercy of an environment over which they have little control. Food is limited, death rates are high and life is short, and a species survives only because the deaths are more than offset by an excess in the number of births. It is a picture which Malthus and Darwin would have recognized, memorably described by George Meredith in his poem *Modern Love*.

'I play for Seasons; not Eternities!'
Says Nature, laughing on her way. 'So must
All those whose stake is nothing more than dust!'

And lo, she wins, and of her harmonies
She is full sure! Upon her dying rose,
She drops a look of fondness, and goes by,
Scarce any retrospection in her eye;
For she the laws of growth most deeply knows,
Whose hands bear, here, a seed-bag – there, an urn.

The evidence presented by television suggests that the conditions of human life before the historical period were essentially the same as those of wild animals. Both the external environment and the rate of reproduction appear to have been virtually uncontrolled, and it was the urn which removed the excesses and corrected the errors committed by the seed-bag. In the remarkable panorama, *Life on Earth*, David Attenborough examined communities which still live by hunting and gathering and concluded:

They all live in harmony with the natural world around them, altering it not at all and making do with what it immediately provides. Nowhere are they over-whelmingly numerous. Their expectation of life is short, their birth-rate and the survival of their children are curbed by the scarcity of food and the hazards of their lives. Such was the condition of man for almost all his existence. It is very close to the way in which Upright Man lived about a million years ago. And for about nine hundred and ninety thousand years afterwards, it was the life that he and his descendant, Homo sapiens, was to follow. [1]

It will no doubt come as a surprise to many people to be told that this description of the conditions under which our ancestors evolved is by no means universally accepted. On a few points there is general agreement: that early man was small in stature; that life was short; and that population growth was very slow. But some observers of the few remaining hunter-gatherers have concluded that, far from being at the mercy of a hostile environment, they are, in general, remarkably healthy. The habitat is said to provide a rich supply of plant and animal foods, so that a few hours of gathering by the women and pleasurable hunting by the men are sufficient to ensure that they are well fed. Indeed some enthusiasts give the impression that hunter-gatherers lived an almost idyllic life, from which, initially at least, the change to an agricultural existence can only be regarded as a retrograde step. This conclusion rests, of course, on the beliefs that early man, if unable to control his environment, at least did not waste it; and, even more important, that by restricting fertility and eliminating unwanted births he was able to keep numbers within the limits that the resources of his habitat could support.

[1] Attenborough, D. *Life on Earth*. London, Collins, 1979: 305.

In this interpretation we are at once confronted by some inconsistencies. If early man had an ample and nutritious diet, why was he physically small? If he was healthy, why was life short and mortality high? Above all, how was he able to achieve the critical balance between population size and the resources of the environment which still eludes the people of many countries in the present day?

These questions take us to the heart of the controversy concerning the early history of human health and population growth. The central issue may be stated in this way: At what stage of his existence did man begin to control his environment and limit his numbers to an extent that enabled him to advance his health significantly? On one view, this stage was reached before or soon after the appearance of modern man, about 45,000 years ago. On the other view, the advances were delayed until the historical period, substantial environmental control beginning 10,000 years ago, at or just before the agricultural revolution, and effective limitation of numbers only in the last few centuries. To assess these interpretations we will need to examine the conditions of life and behaviour of early man, particularly in relation to the critical issues of health and population growth.

Human Origins

Although many questions concerning human origins are still unanswered, the main outline is not in doubt. Several million years ago, forest-living apes descended to the plains and gradually became adapted to a new way of life. They are referred to as Australopithecines. In time *Australopithecus* evolved into *Homo erectus*, the ancestor of modern man.

Australopithecines

Ten million years ago apes were widespread in Africa, Europe and Asia. The time of their descent to the plains is unknown, for there are few fossil traces and no humanized remains for the period between 10 and 4 million years; but from genetic similarities between man and African apes it is believed that the evolutionary division probably occurred about 6 million years ago. From 4 million years the fossil record improves, and it shows that plain-living apes were well established in Africa at that time.

The adaptation from forest to plain life required both physical and physiological changes: to an upright posture, to bi-pedalism; to reliance on sight more than smell; and to the use of the hands for complex tasks. However, the brain of Australopithecines was little larger than that of the apes, and most of the abilities which distinguished their human descendants – the use of tools and fire, cooperative hunting and speech – were still beyond them.

Homo erectus

Two million years ago, early stone tools were in use, and the human ancestor at this stage is referred to as *Homo habilis*. His brain was not much larger than that of the ape; but it increased fairly rapidly in size, and at 1.6 million years, when *Homo erectus* is identified, it had almost doubled. The reasons for the enlargement are not clear; it was once thought to have resulted from bi-pedalism or the freeing of the hands, but this is now considered unlikely. Speech, if present, was still in a primitive form.

Homo erectus was a successful competitor for the plant and animal foods of the savannah, and was fortunate in having no natural predators. Numbers increased, and in time he spread from Africa to the Nile Valley, the Eastern Mediterranean and Europe. He is also known to have existed in the Far East – bones have been discovered in Java and China – either as a result of migration from Africa or from independent origins. This worldwide migration took *Homo erectus* into conditions very different from those in which his ape-like ancestors had evolved; but he learned to protect himself against the hazards and in time his body and ways of life became adapted to the new conditions.

Modern Man

There is a fairly continuous fossil record from *Homo erectus* to modern man. Remains of a form intermediate between the two have been found as far apart as Britain and China, but it is uncertain whether the evolution occurred in one place – Africa, or possibly Europe or West Asia – or in several places independently. *Homo sapiens* is identified from 600,000 years ago, about the time when the use of fire was discovered; except for this advance basic skills were not much greater than those of *Homo erectus*. However, by 100,000 years, when archaic *Homo sapiens* merges into Neanderthal man, cooperative hunting was practised, and there was further evidence of social progress in the burial of the dead and of technical progress in the use of tools, fire and skin clothing. Whether Neanderthals were ancestors of modern (Cro-Magnon) man is still undecided; but as both were well established 34,000 years ago this seems unlikely. From that time at least, speech is believed to have been well developed.

Conditions of Life

Terrain

The ape man, Australopithecus, was ill equipped for extreme climatic conditions, and is believed to have been confined to Africa, or, if there were independent origins in Asia, to tropical and sub-tropical areas. His successors were much more versatile, and from the time of the appearance of *Homo erectus* there was a large extension of the geographical range in Asia and from Africa to Europe. However, fire, clothing and other techniques needed for survival in cold climates had not been discovered, and *Homo erectus* is estimated to have occupied an area roughly equivalent to the Old World south of latitude 50 north, excluding Australia. About a quarter of this area was habitable.

The extension to nearly all other parts of the habitable earth occurred during the Pleistocene epoch, which began about 700,000 years ago and ended not long before the beginning of agriculture. This era more or less coincided with the great Ice Age, in which there were four periods of glaciation separated by three interglacial intervals. In the cold periods the polar ice cap covered northern Europe, northern Asia, most of Canada and all of England and Wales; in the warmer intervals the temperature rose and forests again invaded the arctic tundra.

Not long after the beginning of the Ice Age, *Homo sapiens* – as by then he was – acquired the skills that made it possible to live under Arctic conditions, particularly the ability to keep warm and to obtain food: fire was known at least 600,000 years ago; skins of furred animals were used for clothing; caves provided shelter; fish were caught with bone harpoons and wild animals with stone-tipped spears. Indeed in the tundra 'man found an unoccupied ecological niche with abundant resources and no other major predator except wolves, and with a challenge which his high intelligence enabled him to exploit'.[2]

The ability to live under arctic conditions enlarged the human habitat; it was extended still further when, as the ice cap retreated, hunters entered the Arctic Circle and discovered in the Bering Strait the land bridge which at times during the Ice Age linked Asia and North America. So at a comparatively late date, some time between 25,000 and 10,000 BC, man entered the Americas, quite unaware that he now had access to the space and resources of two continents. Much earlier, by way of the Indonesian archipelago, he had discovered Australia, so that by the end of the

[2] Fiennes, R. N. *Zoonoses and the Origins and Ecology of Human Disease*. London, Academic Press, 1978: 3.

Pleistocene period almost the whole of the habitable world was thinly occupied.[3]

Social Organization

In relation to the health of hunter-gatherers, the most significant conclusions about their ways of life are that they lived in conditions which minimized exposure to human infections, and that they neither eroded nor substantially improved their physical environment.

Present-day hunters live in small groups, normally of twenty-five to fifty people, sometimes fewer but rarely about one hundred. Infrequently, when food is plentiful, they make contact with larger groups, but in a lifetime an individual is unlikely to see more than a few hundred people. In Palaeolithic times population densities must have varied considerably, but they were always low, rarely above a few persons per square mile. It would be difficult to describe conditions less suitable for the establishment of human infectious organisms which have no other animal host.

Hunter-gatherers were nomads, moving about a loosely defined territory in small familial groups in search of food. For much of the year they had no settled abodes, but where climate was unfavourable they made use at times of caves and simple dwellings. Fiennes has noted that this life-style is 'strikingly similar to that of man's fellow tundra predators, the wolves, which live in small family groups in insanitary dens during the summer and follow the wildlife migration in larger packs during the winter'.[4]

Food was obtained from hunting by the men and gathering by the women, and, as noted below, the balance between the two varied widely from place to place. What is significant in the present context is that the methods used – hunting and fishing by simple means and the gathering of roots, seeds, fruit and nuts that grew naturally – neither wasted nor significantly improved the environment. An economy of this kind would not deteriorate, and could meet indefinitely the needs of the people it could support; but it could not expand, and when population size exceeded the tolerable limits it would be necessary to seek food in other areas. This in essence is the history of land use in the Pleistocene epoch, when there was neither erosion of food sources nor sufficient control of the environment to make it possible substantially to increase them.

Food

The earliest mammals were insectivores, and invertebrate predation was the basis from which primate feeding evolved. 'However as the primate

[3] McEvedy, C. and Jones, R. *Atlas of World Population*. London, Penguin, 1985: 13, 14.
[4] Fiennes, R. N. *Zoonoses*: 8.

order expanded and body size increased, vegetable foods became increasingly important. During the Miocene era (from about 24 to 5 million years ago) fruits appear to have been the main dietary constituent for hominids, but their fossilized dental remains seem suitable for mastication of both animal and vegetable material'.[5] The diets of present-day wild primates are extremely varied: an examination of 55 genera showed that 32 have natural diets that include plant and animals foods, 16 are vegetarians whose diets consist of herbaceous materials and fruits, and 4 are carnivorous. The variation in feeding habits is well illustrated by the diets of some of the primates close to the ancestors of early man: the Orangs and the Gibbons are fruit eaters; gorillas are pure herbivores, and subsist mainly on fruit and leaves that can be reached from the ground; chimpanzees are omnivorous, and in addition to fruit and vegetables eat insects, honey, birds' eggs and small mammals.[6]

Against this background of experience of his primate ancestors, it is not surprising that man was able to adapt his eating habits to the varied foods available in different parts of the world. He lacked the gorilla's ability to digest vegetation in its most abundant forms, as leaves and grasses; but eventually the deficiency was more than compensated for by his ability to hunt, to cultivate and to employ the cow and the goat to digest the indigestible for him.

The food of early man was predominantly vegetarian, supplemented, like that of the chimpanzee, with insects and small animals that were readily available. The diets were probably characterized, like those of some present-day hunter-gatherers, by the large number of food items: Lee estimated that Kung Bushmen eat 85 species of plants and 54 species of animals, although only 9 of the plant species are eaten in large amounts and 17 of the animals are consistently hunted.[7] With the development of better tools and more skilful hunting, the amount of meat increased. The use of aquatic foods is a relatively recent development, however, as shells and fish bones are not found in archaeological material dating before 130,000 years ago and are infrequent before 20,000 years ago. It is believed that *Homo erectus* and early *Homo sapiens* obtained the bulk of their food from plant sources.[8]

The variation in diets of hunter-gatherers is well illustrated by observations on the handful of hunters who survive today. Most live in semi-tropical areas and obtain between 50 and 80 per cent of their food

[5] Eaton, S. B. and Konner, M. 'Palaeolithic nutrition.' *N. Eng. J. Med.*, 1985 **312**: 283-9.

[6] Attenborough, D. *Life on Earth*: 291.

[7] Truswell, A. and Truswell, S. 'Diet and nutrition of hunter-gatherers.' In: *Health and Disease in Tribal Societies*. London, CIBA Foundation Symposium, **49** (new series), 1977: 213-21.

[8] Eaton, S. B. and Konner, M. Palaeolithic nutrition.

from plants. Within these limits there is considerable variation: the Hadza
of Tanzania, for example, have 20 per cent of their diet from animal food,
whereas some groups of Australian Aborigines have between 37 and 97 per
cent from meat or fish.[9] People living near seas and rivers obtain a
considerable proportion of their food from fish and shellfish, and the
Eskimos, for whom vegetable foods are rarely available, are almost entirely
carnivorous.

In their appraisal of the Palaeolithic diet, Eaton and Konner noted that
the foods we eat today are divided into four basic groups: meat and fish;
vegetables and fruit; milk and milk products; and bread and cereals. Early
man had no dairy products, and was rarely able to consume cereal grains.
On the average, and subject to wide variation, the diet consisted of about
35 per cent meat; the rest came from vegetable sources.[10]

But although there is broad agreement about the kinds of food eaten by
early man, the most important question remains unanswered: Was there
enough of it? I shall return to this question when considering the health and
disease of hunter-gatherers.

In his search for food man covered most of the earth; he was ready to
submit to inhospitable conditions and to adapt his eating habits to the
diverse materials that were available. Was the adaptation mainly cultural
or genetic? Writing of the Kalahari Bushmen Tobias stated:

It is not the slow cultural genetic adjustment nor the smooth and reversible
functional accommodation but the swift, intelligent cultural adaptation which has
permitted the Bushmen to cope with the rigours of his environment. It is remarkable
that even in a pre-neolithic economy like that of the Bushmen, culture predominates
over biological considerations in ensuring survival.[11]

And Barnes noted that:

while Eskimos have certain genetic traits such as facial hairlessness and narrow
noses, which are advantageous in arctic conditions, it is nevertheless their complex
cultural inventions that enable them to live as hunters on the border of the habitable
world.[12]

According to these views, if Eskimos and Bushmen were to exchange
habitats, their difficulties in the new terrains would owe more to their

[9] Barnes, F. 'The biology of pre-neolithic man.' In: Boyden, S. V. (ed.) *The Impact of
Civilisation on the Biology of Man*. Canberra, Australia National University Press, 1970: 1–18.
[10] Eaton, S. B. and Konner, M. Palaeolithic nutrition.
[11] Tobias, P. V. 'Bushman hunter-gatherers: a study in human ecology.' In: Davis, D. H.
S. (ed.) *Ecological Studies in Southern Africa*. The Hague, W. Junk, 1964: 67–86.
[12] Barnes, F. Biology of pre-neolithic man.

cultural than to their physiological deficiencies. I can well believe it, having once observed two French-speaking black Africans in a restaurant at Lagos where their plane had made an unscheduled stop. When told that for lunch they could have only the traditional British fare – meat, two vegetables and no wine – their speech, gestures, and facial expressions were precisely those of two Frenchmen who had crossed the Channel and faced the barbarities of the English cuisine for the first time.

Population Size And Restraints On Its Increase

In the debate on the health of hunter-gatherers, some of the most fundamental questions concern the nature and effectiveness of restraints on population growth. The slow increase of numbers over a long period leaves no doubt that growth was retarded; but in relation to the resources available was it limited by mains and to an extent consistent with the requirements of health?

As the population of the world before the nineteenth century is unknown, and even today is subject to an error of at least 10 per cent, all calculations for the prehistoric period are from indirect sources and must be offered with reservations. The numbers of great apes have been used as indications of lower and upper limits of the Australopithecine population of two to three million years ago: it is estimated that there are almost 70,000 gorillas with a density of one per km. and more than one million chimpanzees with a density of three to four per km. When *Homo erectus* spread widely from Africa to other continents numbers undoubtedly increased, to perhaps 1.7 million, at a density of 1 per 10 km. or 2 to 3 per 100 km. of habitable terrain. This density is much lower than that of gorillas, which are of comparable size, but the difference is said to be explained by man's inability to digest vegetable foods such as leaves and grasses, and his greater dependence on less readily available meat and other foods. These population estimates for *Homo erectus* are roughly consistent with those for some present-day populations, such as the aborigines of Australia, who live in comparable conditions.

Numbers of *Homo sapiens* are thought to have been of the same order, although they may have contracted somewhat during the Ice Age when arctic conditions reduced the habitable area. But when our ancestors reached Australia by way of Indonesia and crossed the Bering Strait into the Americas, the amount of habitable land was vastly increased. The population again expanded, and by 10,000 BC, just before the Agricultural Revolution, it is thought to have been about 4 million. This is a considerable advance from the 1.7 million of *Homo erectus*; but it occurred over a period of more than a million years, and when compared with population growth rates of the past few centuries it is a very slow rate of increase. That there must have been restraints on numbers is one of the few major conclusions on health and population growth of early man about which there is no serious disagreement. The differences of opinion arise in relation to the nature and extent of the restraints with, as we shall see, large implications for conclusions on health in the prehistoric period.

The reasons for the slow growth of the human population are usually discussed in terms of low fertility and high mortality, manifested in either or both a low birth rate and high death rate. However, in relation to health it will be more instructive to distinguish restraints according to whether they were consciously or unconsciously applied. Broadly, this distinction is between measures deliberately taken, such as abortion and infanticide, and those imposed by conditions of life, such as disease and starvation. The former are consistent with health, although not, of course, with the health of the aborted foetus or dead infant; the latter are not.

Deliberate Restraints

It has been suggested that for both early and modern man, deliberate restriction of fertility played an important part in preserving health by limiting population growth to a level consistent with the available resources. This idea is thought to find support in the suggestion, persuasively argued by Wynn-Edwards, that restraints on fertility are common in other animals in their natural habitats, where they maintain 'numbers at about the level at which food resources are utilized to the fullest extent possible without depletion.'[13] The regulation of numbers by behaviour is said to have evolved through group selection, it being to the advantage of a group not to expand beyond its food supplies. This thesis has been criticized on the grounds that natural selection acts by favouring some individuals rather than others and not some populations rather than others, and Lack provided a forceful account of objections to the concept of group selection based on restriction of fertility.[14]

As regulators of numbers, deliberate restraints may be applied before, during or after pregnancy. Needless to say there are no satisfactory data, one might almost say there are no data, on these practices by early man, and conclusions must be drawn from evidence for the historical period, most of it from the present day.

It has been suggested that in the past fertility was limited in various ways

[13] Wynne-Edwards, V. C. *Animal Dispersion in Relation to Social Behaviour*. Edinburgh, Oliver and Boyd, 1972.

[14] Lack, D. *Population Studies of Birds*. Oxford, Clarendon Press, 1966: 299–312.

which reduce the frequency of conception, particularly by avoidance of intercourse, contraconception, sexual taboos and prolonged lactation. There is no convincing evidence that the growth of populations has been limited substantially by deliberate reduction of the frequency of intercourse. Individuals and groups have undoubtedly prevented pregnancy by coitus interruptus and other contraceptive methods, but the earliest indication that they did so on a scale which affected population fertility trends is the decline of the French birth rate from the late eighteenth century. Taboos such as avoidance of intercourse for a time after a birth in association with polygamy may have had some effect; but it is difficult to believe that such practices, provided for primitive people the invaluable capacity to control numbers, and were lost only in the last few centuries since industrialization. There is no evidence of them in the high birth rates of many contemporary developing countries.

The method of reducing fertility on which there is considerable evidence is prolonged lactation, often cited as an effective influence on population growth. When children are breast-fed for long periods it is in order to feed them, rather than to prevent conception, and the effect on fertility is probably small. Thirty per cent of a group of postpartum women became pregnant within a year after delivery; two-fifths of them were still lactating at the time of conception and one-tenth conceived without having menstruated.[15] In another study, the cycle reappeared within five months of birth in forty per cent of mothers whose children were wholly breast-fed. It was concluded that in women, as in experimental animals, the cycle is fairly effectively suppressed during the early period of lactation; it reappears in an increasing proportion as lactation continues, and returns more rapidly if the child is partially weaned.[16] Moreover, the ability of the breast to secrete enough milk to feed a child diminishes after the early months, and children kept at the breast for the long periods quoted for primitive people, if they are not grossly underfed, must be receiving their food largely from other sources. Under such conditions the stimulus of suckling is reduced and the effect on fertility is small, for it is suckling that inhibits the sexual cycle.

Fertility may also be reduced by termination of pregnancies by abortion. Recent experience (for example in Japan and Britain) leaves no doubt about the effectiveness of abortion, and the only question is whether it was successful with the techniques available before the twentieth century. There is no reason to think so. In spite of the extensive lore about abortion

[15] Peckham, C. G. 'An investigation of some effects of pregnancy noted six weeks and one year after delivery.' *Bulletin, Johns Hopkins Hospital,* 1934, **54**: 186.

[16] McKeown, T. and Gibson, J. R. 'A note on menstruation and conception during lactation.' *Journal of Obstetrics and Gynaecology of the British Empire,* 1954, **61**: 824.

produced by drugs, violence and psychological stress, it is difficult to interrupt a normal pregnancy by any means other than direct interference with the contents of the uterus. (Sarah Gamp, Dickens' garrulous midwife in *Martin Chuzzlewit*, was mistaken in saying of pregnant women that 'little puts us out . . . a chimbley sweep, a newfundlanddog, or a drunkin man a-coming round the corner sharp, may do it'). An abortion can be induced with reasonable safety by an experienced physician operating under hygienic conditions. In any other circumstances the procedure is both unreliable and dangerous, and often results in the septic complications which were common in hospitals before the grounds for abortion were liberalized. In most cases they were caused by passing instruments of various kinds through the cervix into the uterus. It is inconceivable that abortion could have provided for early man what it has not until recently provided for modern man, a safe and effective means of restricting fertility.

But whatever doubts there may be about the control of fertility, there is no reason to question that numbers were substantially reduced by deliberate killing or neglect of unwanted individuals after birth. The importance of the different methods – infanticide, human sacrifice, cannibalism, tribal wars, geronticide – probably varied with time and place; but overall, the most important restraint on population growth was probably from infanticide.

Estimates have been made of its frequency. Birdsell suggested that:

systematic infanticide has been a necessary procedure for spacing human children presumably beginning after man's entry into the niche of bipedalism and lasting until the development of advanced agriculture. It involved between 15 and 50 per cent of the total number of births. Among recent hunters it tends to be preferentially female in character and probably was in the Pleistocene.[17]

For present-day hunter-gatherers Neel reported 25 per cent for females and 15 per cent for both sexes in Amerindians,[18] and Rasmussen counted 38 girls killed out of 96 births in Netsilik Eskimos.[19] There is a great deal of evidence, summarized by Langer, that infanticide was practised on a large scale in both ancient and modern times, and diminished only in the nineteenth century when birth rates declined and conditions of mothers and

[17] Birdsell, J. B. Some predictions for the Pleistocene based on equilibrium systems among recent hunter-gatherers.' In: Lee, R. W. and DeVore, I. (eds) *Man the Hunter*. Chicago, Aldine-Atherton, 1968: 229–40.

[18] Neel, J. V. 'Health and disease in unacculturated Amerindian populations.' In: *Health and Disease in Tribal Societies*. London, CIBA Foundation Symposium **49** (new series), 1977: 155–68.

[19] Rasmussen, K. 'The Netsilik Eskimos: social life and spiritual culture.' *Report of the Fifth Thule Expedition, 1921-1924*, **8**: 1, 2, Copenhagen, Gyldendalske Boghandel, 1931.

children began to improve.[20] It is probable that it persists today, through neglect if not overt killing, particularly in countries where child mortality is high and the survival of male children is considered desirable. Some years ago in a developing country I attended three seminars concerned with the health problems of families. The numbers of surviving children in the families discussed were 19 boys and 2 girls. This remarkable sex ratio was almost certainly due to a high level of female infanticide and passed, I may say, without comment from our hosts. More recently in Britain an experienced obstetrician told me that the same attitude to female births is sometimes seen in the disappointment of a mother when told that her newborn child is a girl.

It is worth noting that experience of infanticide is more consistent with the concept of individual rather than group selection. According to Woodburn 'decisions appear to be made right within the family, often by the mother alone', and 'the making of the choice is relative to the circumstance of a particular mother and not necessarily to the whole population'.[21]

As it was common practice to eliminate a substantial proportion of normal children, it must have been even more usual to kill or neglect those who were handicapped in various ways – by malformation, disease, injury or even by birth as twins. Equally severe treatment was no doubt accorded to individuals whose health or performance was reduced in later life, by disease, injury and infirmity from old age: suicide in crisis situations, invalidicide and senilicide were additional responses to harsh pressures.[22] In respect of hunters in general Coon wrote:

The practice of abandoning the hopelessly ill and aged has been observed in many parts of the world. It has always been done by people in poor environments where it is necessary to move about frequently to obtain food, where food is scarce and transportation difficult. . . . Among peoples who are forced to live in this way the oldest generation, the generation of individuals who have passed their physical peak is reduced in numbers and influence. There is no body of elders to hand on tradition and control the affairs of younger men and women, and no formal system of age grading.[23]

It is difficult to assess the impact of tribal wars or other forms of mass killing. Man is one of the rare species which kill their own kind; most

[20] Langer, W. L. 'Infanticide: A historical survey.' *History of Childhood Quarterly*, 1974, **I**: 353.

[21] Woodburn, J. C. In: Lee, R. W. and DeVore, I. (eds) *Man the Hunter*. Chicago, Aldine-Atherton, 1968: 243.

[22] Balikci, A. 'Quelques cas de suicide parmi les esquimaux Netsilik.' *Actes du VI Congres International des Sciences Anthropologiques et Ethologiques*. Paris, 1960 **2**: 511–16.

[23] Coon, C. S. *Reader in General Anthropology*. New York, Henry Holt, 1948.

animals are able to sublimate their aggressive instincts by ritualized behaviour, by submissive gestures of the weaker which inhibit the stronger from further attack, as in the case of wolves, or by concession of female access or territorial dominance by the weaker to the stronger, as in the case of deer.[24] By comparison with other carnivores human beings are poorly equipped for physical aggression, but even in Palaeolithic times the ability to make and use primitive weapons more than compensated for the deficiency. In some present-day hunter-gatherer societies the killing of one of the group is said to be almost inconceivable, although it has occasionally been reported, usually on a small scale. Its frequency and effects during the Pleistocene are unknown. But if we may extrapolate backwards (very doubtfully) from human behaviour in the historical period, although tribal wars may at times have had a devastating effect in limited areas, overall they probably had much less influence on population growth than the elimination of a substantial proportion of all children by infanticide soon after birth. The same may be said about hunting accidents, also thought to have contributed significantly through injury and wound infection.

Unconscious Restraints

Although there are differences of opinion about the relative effectiveness of control of fertility and postnatal killing, it is generally agreed that deliberate restraints had a considerable effect on population growth. But were they able to keep numbers within the limits determined by the resources of the environment, so that unconscious restraints which prejudiced health were not imposed by starvation, malnutrition and disease? In spite of the apparent ease of living of some present-day hunters, and recognizing the deficiencies of the evidence, for the following reasons I conclude that the control of numbers was insufficient.

1   The observations on present-day hunter-gatherers are by no means consistent. Those who have abundant food supplies are matched by others who work hard for their food and are often hungry.[25] These differences of conditions among the few remaining hunters suggest, as would surely be expected, that the resources of our Pleistocene ancestors varied greatly from time to time and from place to place.

2   The fact that *Homo erectus* spread widely to all parts of the Earth which could conceivably support human life, even under the most severe conditions, suggests that food resources generally were inadequate and that there was constant pressure to seek to improve them.

24 Barnes, F. Biology of pre-neolithic man.
25 Lee, R. W. and DeVore, I. (eds) 'Problems in the study of hunters and gatherers.' In: *Man the Hunter*, Chicago, Aldine-Atherton, 1968: 3–12.

3   The ability to equate numbers and resources, if it existed, must have been deeply rooted in instinctive behaviour. It is difficult to believe that it would have been lost in a few generations, as a result of the changes to agricultural and industrial life.

4   I have concluded that infanticide was probably the most effective deliberate influence on control of numbers. It is hard to believe that mothers would consent to kill or abandon their children while food supplies were adequate. They (unlike fathers) did not do so in Hiroshima and Nagasaki under some of the most stressful conditions to which human beings have ever been exposed.

5   If numbers had been kept below the limits imposed by the food resources of the environment, the effects of natural selection would have been greatly reduced, and some differences between races in body structure and physiology would not have occurred.

On the last point: the conclusion that control of numbers would have reduced the effects of natural selection is based on the fact that deliberate restraints are essentially random in their effects. This is certainly true of methods of reducing fertility: taboos on sexual intercourse, contraception and abortion are all genetically unselective; it is only recently, and to a trivial extent, that contraception and abortion have been practised in ways which might affect the genetic composition of a population. Infanticide was clearly a random procedure, determined largely by considerations – sex of offspring, family size and availability of food – unrelated to genes. Killing or neglect of aged people would have little or no selective effects, and only the elimination early in life of those handicapped by disease or malformation might have had some influence. However, since few congenital abnormalities are determined irreversibly at fertilization, the effects from the early deaths of those affected would be very small.

I conclude that although deliberate restraints on population size were widely practised, and at certain times and places may have kept numbers within limits imposed by the resources of the environment, in general they were unable to do this, and the expansion of populations was restricted substantially by mortality due to external causes such as starvation, malnutrition and disease.

Health and Disease

As there is no direct information about human health during the Pleistocene, conclusions are necessarily based on evidence from three sources: observations of other animals, particularly primates, in their natural habitats; archaeological evidence; and investigations of conditions of life and health of the few hunter-gatherers who still exist. All of this evidence is indirect and incomplete, so it is essential to evaluate it in the light of current knowledge and experience.

Other Animals

To throw light on the problems of human disease in the hunter-gatherer period, what is needed for other animals is evidence, particularly quantitative evidence, of their disease experience when living in their natural habitats. Unfortunately this information is rarely available. The observations that have been made are chiefly on animals domesticated, in zoos or, if free living, affected in various ways by the man-made environment; disease reports on wild animals are usually based on single or few specimens and without knowledge of the size of the populations from which they are drawn. But although it is not possible to make estimates of disease frequency or to assess accurately the relative importance of different causes of death, some general conclusions have been drawn.

First, many ecologists are agreed that 'in populations of wild animals, disease is of rather secondary importance in population control, and only becomes of significance when population pressure becomes so heavy that the animals lose their natural resistance to parasites.'[26, 27] Second, the disease which occurs is predominantly due to infection caused by parasites; indeed symposia on disease in free-living wild animals have been devoted almost exclusively to infectious diseases.[28] Third, although non-communicable diseases do occur in animals affected by the man-made environment, in the wild they are very uncommon, particularly in primates.

Because of its bearing on the problems of human health, the evidence on which the last conclusion is based is of great interest, particularly in relation to the most common causes of death in developed countries, cardiovascular disease and cancer. There have been scattered reports of sclerotic vascular lesions in wild animals, but only the pig, the whale and possibly some non-human primates have been observed to develop a 'spontaneously' progressive disease which resembles human atherosclerosis.[29] In primates, systematic studies have been made in baboons, rhesus monkeys and squirrel monkeys. They suggest that hypertension and atherosclerotic

26 Fiennes, R. N. *The Environment of Man*. London, Croom Helm, 1978: 18.

27 Fiennes, R. N. 'Stress and diseases of the cardiovascular system.' In: Hoff, G. L. and Davis, J. W. (eds) Iowa, Iowa State University Press, 1982: 58.

28 McDiarmid, A. (ed.) *Diseases in Free-Living Wild Animals*. Symposia of the Zoological Society of London, **24**, London, Academic Press, 1969.

29 Roberts, J. C. and Strauss, R. (eds) *Comparative Atherosclerosia*. New York, Harper and Row, 1965.

changes (not affecting the cerebral or cardiac vessels) are sometimes seen in monkeys used in experiments and kept in regular cages over long periods; they are rarely seen in animals kept in open-air cages and 'there is no direct reference in the literature to the possibility of atherosclerosis developing in monkeys in their natural habitats.'[30] The complications of atherosclerosis – thrombosis, aneurysm and myocardial infarction – are very uncommon,[31] and only five cases of coronary occlusion caused by infarcts have been reported for non-human primates. From their extensive study of the pathology of Rhesus monkeys, Lapin and Yakovleva concluded that 'coronary insufficiency is rightly considered a disease seen only in man'.[32]

So far as it goes, the evidence suggests that spontaneous tumours of free-living wild animals are also rare. Knowledge of tumours, as indeed of most diseases of wild animals, is derived from observations on animals kept in the unnatural environments of breeding farms and zoos. Even under such conditions tumours, both benign and malignant, are very uncommon in primates and they seldom metastasize. Fiennes noted that before 1972 'only some 200 spontaneous tumours had been described in the literature, in spite of the large numbers of monkeys and apes that have been kept in zoos and research establishments'.[33] Moreover, in other mammals, unlike man, the tumours which do occur are believed to be mainly viral in origin. The same is said to be true of plant cancers. Writing more generally of non-communicable diseases in primates, Lapin and Yakovleva concluded that 'the diseases that are most common in man, i.e. malignant neoplasms, rheumatism, cardiovascular diseases, they either occurred seldom or not at all in monkeys'.[34]

The main causes of death of other animals discussed by population biologists are food shortage, predation, parasites and disease, taking parasites to include all infectious agents – viruses, bacteria, protozoa, helminths and arthropods. In this interpretation the distinction between predators and parasites is based on the fact that predators kill by intention and feed on the dead host, whereas parasites feed on the living host and kill only inadvertently. Hence it is to the advantage of the parasite as well as of the host that the host should be healthy; 'the death of the host is a result as harmful to the virus's future as to that of the host itself'.[35]

A further division can be made between micro and macroparasites.

[30] Lapin, B. A. and Yakovleva, L. A. *Comparative Pathology of Monkeys*. Springfield, Thomas, 1963.

[31] Fiennes, R. N. Stress and diseases of the cardiovascular system: 65.

[32] Lapin, B. A. and Yakovleva, L. A. *Comparative Pathology*: 139.

[33] Fiennes, R. N. *Infectious Cancers of Animals and Man*. London, Academic Press, 1982: 79.

[34] Lapin, B. A. and Yakovleva, L. A. *Comparative Pathology*: 254.

[35] Andrewes, C. *Viruses and evolution*. University of Birmingham, The Huxley Lecture, 1965-66.

Microparasites are broadly those having direct reproduction, usually at high rates, within the definitive host, (as typified by most viral and bacterial and many protozoan infections); the duration of infection is usually short, relative to the expected life span of the host, and is therefore of a transient nature. Macroparasites are those having no direct reproduction within the host (as typified by most helminthic infections); infections are usually of a persistent nature, with hosts being continually reinfected.[36]

The evidence summarized above suggests that non-communicable disease is·a very uncommon cause of death of wild animals, so that the causes to be considered are food shortage, predators, parasites and infectious disease. But the infections are due to parasites as defined above, so that the predominant causes of death are really three.

As there is a large literature on food, infection and predator-prey inter-actions in wild animals, it is perhaps surprising that more attempts have not been made to assess the relative importance of different causes of death. Investigators have no doubt been discouraged by the difficulties, not least by the fact that the causes do not act independently, and several may be involved in the control of numbers, even in a single species.

At first sight the conclusion that disease is of secondary importance in population control (see p. 30) appears to be inconsistent with many well authenticated examples of high mortality from infectious diseases of wild animals. In his review of the literature Holmes noted several references to large-scale epizootics of disease. In waterfowl, among the most intensively studied vertebrates, some were caused by viruses, such as duck viral enteritis in South Dakota where 40,000 mallards died; others were due to bacteria, such as avian cholera in Missouri, where 1100 snow geese died in a single night, or botulism which killed 4–5 million ducks in 1952; still others were from fungi, blood protozoa or nematode infections.[37] Many more examples could be cited in vertebrates, such as the dramatic panzootic of rinderpest that swept through Africa and killed vast numbers of cattle and wild ungulates.

In spite of this evidence, many population biologists are not convinced that infection plays a large part in the regulation of animal numbers, particularly in vertebrates. Although it is sometimes a proximate cause of death, it appears to be a consequence of population size rather than a determinant of it; parasites are generally rare in low density populations. Parasitism is therefore said to act in a compensatory fashion, in the sense

36 May, R. M. 'Introduction.' In: Anderson R. M. and May, R. M. (eds) *Population Biology of Infectious Diseases*. Berlin, Springer-Verlag, 1982: 1–12.

37 Holmes, J. C. 'Impact of infectious disease agents on the population growth and geographical distribution of animals.' In: Anderson, R. M. and May, R. M. (eds) *Population Biology of Infectious Diseases*. Berlin, Springer-Verlag, 1982: 37–51.

that if disease did not occur other causes of death would lead to the same level of mortality. The more fundamental influences, it is suggested, are those with which infection interacts – food shortage, predation, stress, population pressure.

Population pressure is an unsatisfactory term; stress is more accurately defined, but is a response rather than a primary influence; so that we are left with food shortage and predation (including hunting) as clearly defined influences which interact with infection as major causes of death. Lack considered that outside the breeding season starvation is much the most important density-dependent factor in wild birds, and that 'the numbers of certain rodents, large fish where not fished, and a few insects are limited by food'. However, the number of gallinaceous birds, deer and phytophagous insects for most of the time are limited by predators (including insect parasites).[38]

But although the relative importance of food shortage, predation, and disease due to parasites is still debated, there is a way of looking at the problem which leads to a general conclusion. Starvation and malnutrition are due directly to food deficiency. Predators are in search of food, and in some cases are less active if ample supplies of alternative plant foods are available. Parasites feed on their hosts, and cause disease mainly when the host is debilitated, often because it is malnourished.[39, 40] Although it is possible that there are exceptions to this generalization,[41] this does not affect the conclusion that the death of animals in their natural habitats is due mainly to food deficiency, acting directly through starvation and malnutrition, or indirectly through hazards from other living things – predators (including human predators) and parasites – seeking food.

Archaeological Evidence

The materials available to archaeologists from the Palaeolithic are bone and stone, and to understand how little they can contribute to knowledge of the diseases of early man we have only to recognize their limitations. In the first place, examinations of skeletons or bone fragments provide no information about abnormalities which affect only soft tissues, so that observations on the infections are limited to the few diseases, such as

[38] Lack, D. *Population Studies of Birds*: 187, 280.

[39] Allison, A. C. 'Co-evolution between hosts and infectious disease agents and its effects on virulence.' In: Anderson, R. M. and May, R. M. (eds) *Population Biology of Infectious Diseases*. Berlin, Springer-Verlag, 1982: 245–67.

[40] Holmes, J. C. Impact of infectious disease agents.

[41] Levin, B. R. 'Evolution of parasites and hosts group report.' In: Anderson, R. M. and May, R. M. (eds) *Population Biology of Infectious Diseases*. Berlin, Springer-Verlag, 1982: 213–43.

tuberculosis, syphilis and leprosy, which cause changes in bones. Secondly, the specimens examined, often in collections in museums and universities, are relatively small in number and drawn from populations whose size is unknown. Quantitative data are therefore unavailable, and the most that can be said is that abnormalities affecting bones have occurred at times in certain places.

Such information is by no means unimportant. It tells us that tuberculosis probably can be identified from about 3000 BC, leprosy from AD 500 and syphilis from AD 1500.[42] It provides evidence of degenerative bone pathology; Neanderthal man is believed to have suffered frequently from osteoarthritis – arthritic changes were found in seventeen of twenty-seven skeletons from a site in California. In the same series there was also evidence of osteomyelitis, sinusitis and alveolar abscesses, although dental caries is rare in hunter-gatherers.[43] Traumatic lesions are quite common in archaeological material, the site of the injury varying, as might be expected, with the nature of the habitat.

Even less direct evidence on diseases of early man is based on examination of fossils. The absence of eggs of parasitic helminths was said to show that the people represented by the specimens were free of many intestinal helminths, including flukes, tapeworms and nematodes such as hookworm and Ascaris.[44] Perhaps the most satisfactory use of archaeological material has been in determination of foods in common use, since it is possible to excavate both the remains of food and the tools used to obtain it. Even here, however, there is need for caution; plant foods and the tools used in gathering are quite perishable, whereas evidence of hunting is recorded in the more durable materials of bone and stone. The ratio of hunting to gathering may therefore be overestimated.

From the exiguous evidence, archaeologists have concluded cautiously that disease patterns in the past were not markedly different from those of the present day.[45] But they recognize the tentative nature of this conclusion, and that 'it is doubtful whether we shall ever obtain the evidence to confirm our suspicions that the majority of the people who are excavated from their ancient graves were originally laid in them because of infectious diseases'.[46]

[42] Moller-Christensen, V. 'Leprosy and tuberculosis.' In: Hart, G. D. (ed.) *Disease in Ancient Man*. Toronto, Clarke Irwin, 1983: 129–38.

[43] Barnes, F. Biology of pre-neolithic man.

[44] Dunn, F. L. 'Epidemiological factors: health and disease in hunter gatherers.' In: Lee, R. W. and DeVore, I. (eds) *Man the Hunter*. Chicago, Aldine-Atherton, 1968: 221–28.

[45] Dobson, J. 'The medical historian's point of view.' In: Hart, G. D. (ed.) *Disease in Ancient Man*. Toronto, Clarke-Irwin, 1983: 45–9.

[46] Birkett, D. A. 'Non-specific infections.' In: Hart, G. D. (ed.) *Disease in Ancient Man*. Toronto, Clarke-Irwin, 1983: 99–105.

Present-Day Hunter-Gatherers

Until the beginning of agriculture 10,000 years ago, the whole of the world's population subsisted by hunting and gathering. From that time, however, land was gradually converted to agricultural use, about half by the time of Christ and more than three-quarters by the time of the discovery of the New World.[47] Today hunter-gatherers are to be found in only a few isolated pockets, mainly at the centre and periphery of continents. Nevertheless, the first comprehensive survey in 1968 included reports of hunters still living in all continents except Europe.[48]

Because of the paucity of other data on the health of early man, contemporary evidence has been exploited for all, and perhaps occasionally for more than it is worth. It raises two related questions which are difficult to answer: Are present-day hunter-gatherers typical of their Pleistocene ancestors? And to what extent have they been affected by contact with agricultural and, latterly, industrial people?

On the first point: As their numbers have diminished hunter-gatherers have been increasingly restricted to unfavourable land areas, unattractive for agricultural and other uses; Eskimos, Australian aborigines and Kung bushmen once lived in much better habitats than those they now occupy. It is therefore possible that hunters in good environments are most representative of their predecessors. However, many of the less favourable habitats have also been abandoned, so that the change in balance between good and bad environments has not been entirely in one direction.

On the second point: Hunter-gatherers have been affected in various ways by contact with other people. In relation to health perhaps the most significant finding is that they have been exposed to infectious diseases from which formerly they were probably free. Respiratory viruses for example, are not generally carried by normal subjects and cannot persist in small isolated communities:[49] yet the relative isolation of the Bushmen of the Kalahari desert has not protected them from respiratory infections.[50] This evidence of external influences clearly suggests that hunter-gatherers have been affected in other ways which are unrecognized.

In almost every aspect of their lives and health there are different findings and different interpretations. This is not surprising in view of the wide diversity of the conditions under which they live, from the Arctic

[47] Murdock, G. P. 'The current status of the world's hunting and gathering people.' In: Lee, R. W. and Devore, I. (eds) *Man the Hunter*. Chicago, Aldine-Atherton, 1968: 13–20.

[48] Lee, R. W. and DeVore, I. *Man the Hunter*.

[49] Tyrrell, D. A. J. 'Aspects of infection in isolated communities.' In: *Health and Disease in Tribal Societies*. London. CIBA Foundation Symposium **49** (new series) 1977: 137–43.

[50] Brown, P. K. and Taylor-Robinson, D. 'Respiratory virus antibodies in sera of persons living in isolated communities.' *Bull. W. H. O.*, 1966, **34**: 895–900.

Circle to tropical forest lands to the Australian and Kalahari deserts. In his review of health and disease in hunter-gatherers Dunn was understandably sceptical about the possibility of generalizations: 'They are diverse, their hunting territories are diverse, and so are their diseases and ways of death'; and he concluded that 'hunters today do not live in wholly aboriginal or "prehistoric" states of health, and historic or ethnographic records offer little data upon which to base speculations about prehistoric conditions of health.'[51]

There is, perhaps, least disagreement about their experience of non-communicable diseases. Congenital abnormalities are believed to be uncommon, at least in surviving children, as would be expected in nomadic people when serious disability often leads to early death. Many chronic diseases of developed countries – hypertension, cardiovascular disease, cancer, obesity, diabetes, dental caries – are rare or absent, although the interpretation of this finding has been guarded because most hunter-gatherers do not live to the ages at which these diseases are common.[52, 53]

It is generally agreed that trauma is a frequent cause of injury and death but again the causes vary according to the way of life and character of the habitat.

Falls from trees produce injuries amongst the Siriono, fractured arms are found in Aborigines hunting over boulder stream country, while Colles's fracture and fractures of the small bones of the leg occurred in the Californian men gathering seafood on a slippery floor. Drowning is a frequent cause of death among young male Eskimos, while eye injuries from branches are common among Bushmen. Snake bites and attack by predators are significant dangers in some habitats; the latter may have been even more important in early savannah environments.[54]

For a number of reasons it is difficult to make reliable observations on infectious diseases in present-day hunter-gatherers, and still more, to use them as a basis for conclusions about the disease experience of their Pleistocene ancestors. Examination of contemporary populations tells us little about past experience of infection, particularly in those who died at an early age and all present-day hunters appear to have been exposed through outside contacts to infectious diseases which could not have existed under the conditions which prevailed during the Pleistocene.

Lacking data for truly isolated communities, observers have used serological and clinical methods to assess the infections. On the basis of immunological evidence from several investigations, Black concluded that

51 Dunn, F. L. Epidemiological factors.
52 Neel, J. V. Health and disease in Amerindian populations.
53 Dunn, F. L. Epidemiological factors.
54 Barnes, F. Biology of pre-neolithic man.

the diseass of Brazilian Indian tribes fall into four groups:[55] endemic diseases of high incidence and low morbidity (such as herpes and hepatitis B); diseases of low prevalance (such as yellow fever) acquired from other animals; explosive but transient diseases, (such as measles and influenza) introduced from outside the hunter-gatherer communities; persistent diseases (such as tuberculosis and malaria) also introduced from outside. As would be expected, the immunological evidence suggested that the frequency of these diseases varied greatly between tribes.

But perhaps the most inconsistent findings are in respect of food and nutrition. In his appraisal of health and disease in hunter-gatherers, Dunn concluded that malnutrition is rare and starvation occurs only infrequently. Kung bushmen, for example, are reported to live well by a few hours of daily hunting and gathering, and the Hadza of Tanzania are said to be better off than their agricultural neighbours: 'For a Hadza to die of hunger, or even to fail to satisfy his hunger for more than a day or two is almost inconceivable'.[56] But there are exceptions: For some Alaskan Eskimos 'everything is focussed entirely and absolutely upon the requirements that the increasing search for meat necessitates';[57] the Birhor of India not only work hard for their food but often go hungry;[58] and among the Siriono, in the Bolivian rain forest, there appears to be a good deal of hunger which leads to widespread anxiety about food and often to aggressive behaviour. But while recognizing such exceptions, recent writers have emphasized the adequate, sometimes abundant food supplies of hunter-gatherers, and have concluded that the frequency of famine and malnutrition have been exaggerated.

It is from such diverse and inadequate materials that we must try to draw some general conclusions about human health during the Pleistocene. There is least difficulty in the case of non-communicable diseases, since all the evidence points to the same conclusion. Diseases such as cancer, obesity, diabetes, hypertension and heart disease are rare or absent in other primates in their natural habitats; they are very uncommon in present-day hunter-gatherers and peasant agriculturists and only begin to appear when traditional ways of life are abandoned. Indeed it is the observation that primitive societies are largely free from non-communicable diseases which has led to the conclusion that so long as they are undisturbed by external influences, hunter-gatherers remain essentially healthy. There are, however, some exceptions. Archaeological evidence suggests that arthritic conditions were relatively common, and leaves no doubt that trauma was a

[55] Black, F. L. 'Infectious diseases in primitive societies.' *Science*, 1975, **187**: 515–18.

[56] Woodburn, J. C. 'An introduction to Hadza ecology.' In: Lee, R. W. and DeVore, I. (eds) *Man the Hunter*. Chicago, Aldine-Atherton, 1968: 49–55.

[57] Rasmussen, K. Netsilik Eskimos: 142.

[58] Lee, R. W. and DeVore, I. *Man the Hunter*: 3–12.

frequent cause of disability and death. The nature of the injuries varied, as would be expected, with conditions of life, particularly with the means – hunting, fishing, gathering – used to acquire food.

For conclusions concerning infectious diseases we must rely more on insight based on modern knowledge than on observations that have been made, or indeed could be made, on surviving hunter-gatherers. In an illuminating discussion of the infectious diseases of man Fenner wrote: 'In contrast to other types of disease (genetic, traumatic, neoplastic), the infectious diseases are dependent upon contact, either directly or indirectly through fomites, between individuals of the same species or, in the zoonoses, individuals of different species. For this reason social organizations, particularly community size and the degree of frequency of contact between individuals of the same and different communities, has played a significant part in determining the nature and prevalance of the infectious diseases of man.'[59]

As early man lived in small bands with infrequent contact with other closed bands, numbers were not large enough to maintain directly transmitted microparasitic diseases. Under such conditions many of the diseases which were prevalent in the historical period could not have existed: measles, smallpox, whooping cough, poliomyelitis and most enteric and respiratory infections are examples. These diseases are characteristic of generalized human viral infections, for which there is no other animal host and in which latency and recurrent infection does not occur. 'The only "specifically human" viral diseases that we could expect to survive in primitive man are those marked by latency and recurrent disease. Herpes simplex and chickenpox virus, for example, could survive even in isolated family units, because of this characteristic.' Among bacterial and protozoal infections, tuberculosis, leprosy and treponematosis are also diseases from which early man might have suffered, since they are characterized by chronicity and recurrent excretion. Falciparum malaria is believed to have emerged as a human disease in the tropics during the Palaeolithic, but although it may have caused considerable mortality, it is unlikely to have been serious until the development of agriculture led to large populations and conditions suitable for the breeding of mosquito vectors. Fenner considered that cholera was unknown to nomadic Palaeolithic man, but developed when villages and village water supplies were established.[60]

Experience during the Palaeolithic period was quite different in the case of the zoonoses, infections of other animals acquired by direct or indirect

[59] Fenner, F. 'The effects of changing social organisation on the infectious diseases of man.' In: Boyden, S. W. (ed.) *The Impact of Civilization on the Biology of Man.* Toronto: University of Toronto Press, 1970: 48-68.

[60] *Ibid.*

contact or through intermediate hosts. Wild animal reservoirs would have existed for diseases such as brucellosis, leptospirosis, relapsing fever, salmonelloses, tularaemia, mite-born typhus, the rickettsioses and plague. In northern regions wolves become infected with rabies in times of stress when they will attack human beings. In warmer climates man would be exposed to infection by arboviruses carried by primates. Indeed Fenner suggested that jungle yellow fever, mainly a disease of the adult male whose work brings him into close contact with the forest, is a prototype of the sort of viral infection to which Palaeolithic man was exposed.[61] It is anyone's guess how frequently these infections occurred in prehistoric times, and their frequency must have varied widely according to climatic conditions. They were much more common in wet tropics than in deserts.

Finally, hunter-gatherers would have been infected by a group of pathogens referred to as commensals, of which the helminths and other pathogens of the bowel are typical. Most of these organisms are usually harmless, and cause disease only under conditions of stress due to influences such as overcrowding (not a problem for early man) and food-shortage.

I conclude that in spite of occasional dramatic exceptions, early man, like other animals, generally 'lived his life in balance with his pathogens, which only have serious effects at time of ecological imbalance'.[62]

The most controversial question is undoubtedly whether food deficiency was a common cause of sickness and death. It is generally accepted that food supplies set ultimate limits on the size of animal (including human) populations, but it remains in question whether these limits are often reached. After assessing the influences on population growth I concluded that although numbers were deliberately restricted, this occurred under extreme provocation and did not prevent food deficiency.

In summary: For almost the whole of his existence man's ability to control his environment and limit his numbers was insufficient to enable him to advance his health significantly beyond that of other living things. Death rates were high and life was short; but as the number of people born was much greater than the number that survived and reproduced, through natural selection they were well adapted to the conditions under which they lived. The predominant non-communicable diseases of today, such as cancer, heart disease and diabetes, were rare or absent, except for arthritic conditions and disabilities from injuries caused by hunting and other accidents. In the limited sense that they were essentially free from many diseases that are now common, our hunter-gatherer ancestors may be said to have been healthy. It was lack of food, which could not be countered by

[61] *Ibid.*
[62] Fiennes, R. N. *The Environment of Man*: 13.

genetic adaptation, that was chiefly responsible for a high death rate and slow rate of population growth.

Food deficiency limited numbers and prejudiced health in two ways. It led to attempts to restrict population size through reduction of the number of births and by killing or neglecting unwanted individuals. However, the deliberate control of numbers was not sufficient to prevent food shortage, and deaths from starvation, malnutrition and parasitic disease largely associated with poor nutrition were common. Infection was therefore important, although it was not the predominant cause of death that it became in the historical period.

2

Agriculture

The Origins of Agriculture

The first of the two major changes in the conditions of human life occurred in a period of about 8000 years. Until 10,000 years ago all people lived by gathering and hunting the wild plant and animal foods which had fed their ancestors for a few million years; by the time of the birth of Christ nearly everyone lived by farming. This rapid transition raises questions concerning the origins of agriculture which have a considerable bearing on the history of health and population growth.

From the perspective of today it seems almost self-evident that agriculture offered a superior form of life and would be preferred by hunting people as soon as the required technology was available. We therefore tend to think that it was lack of knowledge that delayed its introduction, and that to explain the origins of agriculture we have mainly to account for an advance in understanding of domestication. This approach has indeed been taken, for example by Childe[1] who suggested that in the Middle East, man was brought to a new interest in plants and animals by the drought which occurred at the end of the Pleistocene epoch. Several explanations of this kind have been offered, but most of them depend on local conditions and could hardly explain the widespread transition to agriculture in many parts of the world in a relatively short period.

A more fundamental objection to the idea that agriculture resulted from new advances in technology is the conclusion that much of the knowledge on which it is based was available from early times. Hunter-gatherers knew that plants grow from seeds, and they understand the conditions under which plants and animals thrive. From this knowledge it was not a large step to the control of ecological conditions, and anthropologists have concluded that the distinction between agricultural and pre-agricultural practices is not very great: 'The concept of domestication was not the key

[1] Childe, V. G. *The Prehistory of European Society*. London, Cassell, 1962.

stumbling block in the development of agriculture'.[2] The questions concerning agricultural origins arise in relation to motivation rather than technological knowledge. Why did hunter-gatherers cling for so long to their traditional ways of life if they knew how to replace them? And why did they abandon them at the end of the Pleistocene?

To answer these questions we must leave our present-day perspective and recognize the considerable attractions of the hunting and gathering life. In a symposium on hunting people it was said to be 'the most successful and persistent adaptation man has ever achieved'.[3] Unquestionably it was the most persistent, since it lasted for a few million years; and in many ways it was successful, particularly from the viewpoint of hunters unaware of the attractions of a more sophisticated life. Outside the Arctic, a wide range of plant and animal foods is thought to have provided a diet rich in vitamins, minerals and proteins, sufficient in composition and amount to maintain a healthy population; and because of its variety and inclusion of substantial amounts of meat, the food was more attractive than that of a farmer, based on one or a few cereals. Moreover, there was a degree of security and continuity in the supply that was lost with the advent of agriculture, cultivated crops being more susceptible to climatic influences such as drought. Finally, if experience of present-day hunters can be taken as a guide, it was easier and pleasanter to obtain food by hunting and gathering than by agriculture: 'There is nothing to suggest that people would shift to agriculture to save labour or gain leisure time'. Hence, the question is asked: 'If agriculture provided neither better diet, nor greater dietary reliability, nor greater ease in the food quest; if it did not of itself confer the capability of sedentism, but conversely provided a poorer diet, less reliably, at equal or greater labour costs; why did anyone become a farmer?'[4] If this assessment is accepted, the problem is to explain, not the persistence of hunting and gathering for a few million years, but the reasons for abandoning it in a few thousand.

Against the attractions of the hunter's life, agriculture offered only one advantage, but it was an enormous one; by providing a greater amount of food per unit area of land it could feed a larger population. Agriculture would be likely to be introduced where greater productivity was required, and greater productivity would be needed when population density increased. This conclusion brings us again to the question of the relation between food supplies and population growth, and the issues can be clarified by considering two different interpretations.

According to Malthus, and to those who have adhered to his teaching,

[2] Cohen, M. N. *The Food Crisis in Prehistory*. New Haven, Yale University Press, 1977: 25-6.

[3] Lee, R. B. and DeVore, I. (eds) *Man the Hunter*. Chicago, Aldine-Atherton, 1968: 3.

[4] Cohen, M. N. *Food Crisis*: 39.

variations in population size were determined essentially by the availability of food. When food increased numbers rose and when food decreased numbers fell, because of starvation, malnutrition and disease. This conclusion has much in common with the one reached in chapter 1, and I wish to add only two reservations. Malthus underestimated the effect on population growth of limitation of numbers by methods other than moral restraint; and he had little to say about the possible influence of rising numbers on advances in agricultural technology.

A different explanation of the relation between population growth and technological change was proposed by Boserup, who turned the argument round, making population density the primary influence. She showed that the demands of rising numbers led to advance, not only in agricultural technology, but also in the finance and building of physical and human infrastructure of various types, especially investment in water regulation, energy supply and transportation.[5] One's reservations about this as a general explanation of the relation between technology and population density are that by focussing on technological change as a determinant of food supplies, it understates the importance of food as an influence on population size; and it provides no satisfactory reason for the variation in population density, which Boserup attributed largely to fortuitous changes in mortality from causes such as infectious diseases.[6] Moreover, in relation to the origins of agriculture we must remember that most of the required technology was already available, and it is the decision to apply it that has to be explained.

A plausible explanation was proposed by Cohen,[7] who argued that some common factor is needed to account for the appearance of agriculture within a short period in many different parts of the world. 'The pattern of events for the various regions is consistent with a picture of continuous (although not necessarily steady or consistent) population growth and population pressure'. He suggested that the human population had been growing throughout its history, and that this expansion was a cause rather than merely a result of technological change. For a long time, indeed for a few million years, the needs of the increasing population were largely met within the framework of hunting and gathering, by use of inhospitable land, by acceptance of different and often less palatable food, above all by expansion into new territories. But 'by approximately 11,000 or 12,000 years ago, hunters and gatherers living on a limited range of preferred foods, had by natural population increase and concomitant territorial

[5] Boserup, E. 'The impact of scarcity and plenty on development.' In: Rotberg, R. I. and Rabb, T. K. (eds) *Hunger and History*. Cambridge, Cambridge University Press, 1983: 185–209.

[6] Boserup, E. *Population and Technology*. Oxford, Basil Blackwell, 1981: 36–7.

[7] Cohen, M. N. *Food Crisis*.

expansion fully occupied those portions of the globe which would support their life-style with reasonable ease'. For although hunting and gathering is a successful form of life for small groups, it is not well suited to the support of large or dense populations, and eventually our ancestors 'were forced to adjust to further increases in population by artificially increasing, not those resources which they preferred to eat, but those which responded well to human attention and could be made to produce the greatest number of edible calories per unit of land'.

This explanation is in accord with Malthus' interpretation. It acknowledges attempts to deal with the problem, by reducing demands by limiting number through control of fertility or killing, or by increasing food supplies by resort to different foods and new lands. But although these measures had considerable success, eventually they were insufficient, and it was necessary to seek new methods of production. This explanation reconciles the apparently inconsistent conclusions that increased population density led to technological advance, and that the expansion of population which resulted from the introduction of agriculture was made possible by larger food supplies. To put the matter simply, population pressure led to acceptance of agriculture, but it was agriculture which made it possible to feed much larger numbers.

Health and Disease

The domestication of plants and animals, and the transition from a nomadic to a settled way of life, were the beginning of a degree of control of the environment unique to man. Of the vast changes which resulted from agriculture two were particularly important in relation to health and population growth. One was the increase in food supplies which made possible the expansion of populations. The other was the creation of urban areas with large populations in continuous close contact.

So much attention has been given to the more dramatic episodes in human history that it is not always recognized that for a long time the basic conditions of life remained relatively unchanged. Until the eighteenth century more than 80 per cent of all people lived in rural areas, and as recently as the beginning of the twentieth century Thomas Hardy epitomized the essential features of existence in this way.

> Only a man harrowing clods
> In a slow silent walk
> With an old horse that stumbles and nods
> Half asleep as they stalk.

Only thin smoke without flame
From the heaps of couch grass;
Yet this will go onward the same
Though Dynasties pass.

Although this picture was soon to change in many parts of the world, it is an accurate reflection of conditions in the past. Throughout the agricultural period most people lived on and from the land, experiencing the considerable benefits and associated problems of rural life. Lacking mechanized power they were physically active, assisted in day-to-day labour by domesticated animals; their diet, although different from that of hunter-gatherers, was still based mainly on unrefined plant foods. They were not, in fact, far removed from the conditions for which their genes had equipped them. The chief problem was their poverty, which deprived them of the essentials for life; and the most serious deficiency was in respect of food.

Non-Communicable Diseases

The best evidence on non-communicable diseases comes from a number of studies of peasant agriculturalists who have retained, or only recently changed, their traditional ways of life. In Papua New Guinea, for example, arteriosclerosis and its various manifestations, including coronary heart disease, cerebro-vascular disease and peripheral vascular disease, were rarely seen; obesity, diabetes, hypertension, carcinoma of the bowel and varicose veins were all uncommon. In West Nile Ugandans, blood pressure did not rise with age and essential hypertension and stroke were virtually unknown. Diabetes mellitus was rare in the Bantu rural areas of South Africa and acute appendicitis was not observed in the first thousand Kenyan autopsies. Similar results were obtained in Zimbabwe where coronary thrombosis has only recently appeared in Africans and angina is still a rare disorder.

From these and other observations Trowell and Burkitt constructed a list of non-communicable diseases which appear to be as rare in primitive agriculturalists as in hunter-gatherers. Among medical conditions they included hypertension, obesity, diabetes, gall stones, renal stones and coronary heart disease; and among surgical disorders, appendicitis, haemorrhoids, varicose veins, colo-rectal cancer, hiatus hernia and diverticular disease. Trowell and Burkitt attributed the rarity of these diseases in agriculturalists mainly to their conditions of life, and their increase since the eighteenth century to adoption of the western life-style.[8]

[8] Trowell, H. C. and Burkitt, D. P. (eds) *Western Diseases*. London, Edward Arnold, 1981.

It is in keeping with this interpretation that most of the changes in ways of life from hunting and gathering to agriculture would not be expected to lead to the occurrence of non-communicable diseases. Most people still lived an active rural life, and even the minority living in towns were not exposed to many of the hazards of the present day, such as atmospheric pollution, widespread use of chemicals, adverse working conditions, road traffic, tobacco and drug abuse. The most significant change was in respect of food, which Trowell and Burkitt considered to be the most important of the multiple influences responsible for western diseases in the industrial period.

Under agriculture, there were two important changes in the types of food. Hunter-gatherers lived on meat, fish, fruit and vegetables, and although the proportions of the different foods varied from one population to another, on the average about two-thirds of the diet came from plant sources. They were not often able to have cereals and they had almost no dairy products. Under agriculture man's diet also consisted essentially of vegetable foods, supplemented with meat and fish where these were available. But the common vegetables were cultivated cereals, particularly wheat, rice and maize; wheat accounted for 50 to 70 per cent of the food of those who ate it and rice for 80 to 90 per cent.[9] For some populations dairy products provided a significant part of the diet.

The consumption of cereals did not lead to a substantial increase in the frequency of non-communicable diseases. The vegetables of hunter-gatherers were not limited to those of present-day supermarkets, but included a wide variety of plant foods which contained starch – leaves, fleshy roots, wild berries, wild grass seeds and wild grasses, the precursors of modern wheats. The human body, therefore, had no difficulty in accepting planted and cultivated cereals, since it was well adapted to vegetables with a high proportion of carbohydrates. The problems were to arise later from the introduction of refined and processed foods in which the starch was separated from fibre.

Nevertheless a diet composed mainly of one or a few cereals did expose people from time to time to disease due to deficiencies of proteins, vitamins and minerals. Maize, for example, is short of nicotinic acid which is needed to prevent pellagra; all cereals contain phytate which contributes to rickets because it interferes with the absorption of calcium; and deficiencies may be caused by the preparation of cereals, as in the polishing or rice which reduces the amount of thiamine needed to prevent beri-beri. According to Yudkin, beri-beri, pellagra, riboflavin deficiency and rickets all resulted largely from the dietary changes brought about by the Neolithic revolution.[10] ution.[10]

9 Braudel, F. *The Structures of Everyday Life.* London, Fontana Press, 1985: 145.

10 Yudkin, J. 'Archaeology and the nutritionist.' In: Ucko, P. J. and Dimbley, G. W. (eds) *The Domestication and Exploitation of Plants and Animals.* Chicago, Aldine-Atherton, 1969: 547–52.

The most conspicious deficiency, however, was of certain proteins which led to the disease known as kwashiorkor. This condition was observed in young African children who received little protein in proportion to calories, for example, on a diet comprised of cassava, plaintains, maize meal and little milk. Because of its striking clinical features, kwashiorkor was regarded initially as the most common and severe deficiency disease, but it is now evident that it is much less frequent than disease due to lack of calories, which is less obvious clinically. In a survey in Central America it was found that less than one per cent of children were suffering from severe forms of protein energy malnutrition, but between 50 and 73 per cent had low weight for age. And in India, about one in a hundred children had kwashiorkor, but 80 per cent had reduced growth from an inadequate diet.[11] Most diets which provide enough calories also satisfy protein requirements, and protein deficiency is not a common feature of malnutrition. It would be a useful recognition of this fact if the term protein calorie malnutrition were changed to calorie protein malnutrition.

The other significant change under agriculture was the consumption of dairy products which were not available to hunter-gatherers. Braudel noted wide differences in their use by different populations between the fifteenth and eighteenth centuries. Cheese, milk and eggs were eaten in the West, particularly by the poor for whom they provided an important source of cheap protein. Butter was almost limited to Northern Europe, and its use did not spread until the eighteenth century. In Turkey, milk products were the chief food of the poor, and they were popular throughout Islam as far as the Indies. The striking exceptions were in the vegetarian Far East, where China, Japan and India made little use of dairy products.[12]

It seems unlikely that dairy products could have led to a significant increase in the frequency of cardiovascular disease before the twentieth century. They may have done so in small groups where the intake was excessive, as in East Africa where the wealth of the king and princes of the Wanguana was indicated by the girth of their wives. (In his *Journal of the Discovery of the Source of the Nile* Speke reported that from early youth the women were kept with a pot of milk to their mouths, and some of them 'were fattened to such an extent that they could not stand upright and their flesh hung down like loose stuffed puddings'. It would be surprising if their arteries were not affected.) But excess of this kind was exceptional, for until

[11] Beaton, G. H. and Bengoa, J. M. 'Nutrition and health in perspective: an introduction.' In: Beaton, G. H. and Bengoa, J. M. (eds) *Nutrition in Preventive Medicine: The Major Deficiency Syndrome, Epidemiology and Approaches to Control.* Geneva, World Health Organization, 1971: 45; Gopalan, C. 'Protein versus calories in the treatment of protein calorie malnutrition: metabolic and population studies in India.' In: Olsen, R. E. (ed.) *Protein-Calorie Malnutrition*, London, Academic Press, 1975.

[12] Braudel, F. *Structure of Everyday Life*: 210–13.

the beginning of the twentieth century the consumption of dairy products was severely limited by difficulties of production, preservation and transportation. Indeed, before the discovery of sterilization and pasteurization (about 1900), to obtain milk one had to live within a short distance of a cow or goat, and to obtain safe milk one had to drink it soon after it was produced. As recently as the late nineteenth century cattle were grazed in Hyde Park to provide milk for the population of London. Moreover animals were maintained under more natural conditions than today, and dairy products were not open to some of the objections that have recently been raised.

On the whole, the effects of agriculture on non-communicable diseases were relatively minor, and the really important consequence was the creation of conditions which led to the predominance of infectious diseases as causes of sickness and death.

Infectious Diseases

The importance of infectious diseases in the past is well recognized, and McNeill made a valuable study of their influence at different periods of history.[13] When discussing the infections, however, historians have been more concerned with their effects than with the conditions which led to them, and they sometimes give the impression that their occurrence was largely fortuitous. At first sight this conclusion seems justified, for we are unable to account for day-to-day experience or respiratory and gastrointestinal illnesses, the appearance of influenza cannot be foreseen, and two centuries after the last outbreak of plague in Europe, the reasons for its disappearance are still not entirely clear. Nevertheless, as Fenner noted, social organization has played a major part in determining the nature and prevalence of infectious diseases, and their occurrence in the agricultural and industrial periods can be accounted for largely by the prevailing conditions of life.[14]

There were four main influences which led to the predominance of infectious diseases as causes of sickness and death: the existence, probably for the first time, of populations large enough to enable some human infections to become established and others to be amplified; defective hygiene and crowding, which further increased exposure to communicable diseases; insufficient food which lowered resistance to infection; and close contact with domesticated and other animals which were the probable source of many micro-organisms.

[13] McNeill, W. H. *Plagues and Peoples*. New York. Doubleday, 1976.

[14] Fenner, F. 'The effects of changing social organization on the infectious diseases of man.' In: Boyden, S. F. (ed.) *The Impact of Civilization on the Biology of Man*. Toronto, University of Toronto Press, 1970: 48–68.

Large populations As already noted (see p. 39), early man was exposed to infectious diseases, particularly to the zoonoses, infections of other animals transmitted to man. But living in small groups of no' more than a few hundred persons he must have been free of most human infections, and Burnet considered that under such conditions the infectious diseases which we now know did not exist.

It is generally considered that in the early stages of human evolution primitive man and his subhuman progenitors existed in small wandering groups of at most a few families, and that these groups only rarely come into contact one with the other. Under such circumstances it would be virtually impossible for a pathogen to evolve as a specifically human parasite unless, as in the case of herpes simplex, the period over which a person remains capable of transferring infection was of the order of a generation. . . .

To return to the question of the specifically human virus disease: we have given reasons for believing that in the early phase of human existence, from the beginning of the pleistocene up to about 10,000 years ago, infectious disease due to micro-organisms specifically adapted to the human species was almost non existent. The herpes virus could have persisted with very much its present type of activity, but the viruses producing brief infection with subsequent immunity – measles, mumps and the like – could obviously not have survived in anything like their present form.[15]

The diseases which could not have existed in early man include most of those that were predominant in the historical period. The exceptions, such as herpes simplex and chickenpox among viral diseases, and tuberculosis, leprosy and treponematosis among bacterial and protozoal infections, are characterized by latency and recurrent disease. Their frequency was determined not so much by the human response to the organisms as by hygienic and other conditions which influenced their spread.

By the use of models, Anderson and May have shown that there will be no disease at low levels of vector and host populations unless the efficiency of transmission is very high, as with sexually transmitted diseases.[16] But the situation is different when both populations become large. Various estimates have been made of the size of populations needed to maintain the human infections. According to Cockburn,[17] the first person who considered the significance of population size was Hamer, who wrote in 1906 after a severe influenza epidemic:

[15] Burnet, F. M. *Virus as Organism.* Cambridge, Massachusetts, Harvard University Press, 1946: 30-1.

[16] Anderson, R. M. and May, R. M. 'Directly transmitted infectious diseases: control by vaccination.' *Science*, 1982, **215**: 1053-60.

[17] Cockburn, A. 'Where did our infectious diseases come from? The evolution of infectious disease.' In: *Health and Disease in Tribal Societies.* London, CIBA Foundation Symposium **49**, 1977: 103-12.

It is important to observe that the capacity for smouldering depends upon the existence of a large population densely aggregated. It may be roughly stated that in London, with its 5,000,000 people, some million cases occur up to the time of maximum prevalence; there are after 13 weeks some 5000 cases a week; and a few cases still occur weekly even after six months. On this basis we see that in a population of say 5000 persons, the outbreak would have practically terminated after 13 weeks, and be altogether extinct before the end of half a year. In these considerations we may find explanation for the behaviour of influenza in Martinique, Reunion, or the Fiji Islands.[18]

Table 2.1 Endemicity of measles in islands with populations of 500,000 or less, all of which had at least four exposures to measles during 1949-64

Island	Population	Annual population input*	% months with measles (1949-64)
Hawaii	550,000	16,700	100
Fiji	346,000	13,400	64
Samoa	118,000	4,440	28
Solomon	110,000	4,060	32
French Polynesia	75,000	2,690	8
Guam	63,000	2,200	80
Tonga	57,000	2,040	12
Bermuda	41,000	1,130	51
Gilbert and Ellice	40,000	1,260	15
Cook	16,000	678	6
Falkland	2,500	43	0

* 1956 births less infant mortality.
Source: Fenner, 'The effects of changing social organization on the infectious diseases of man.' In: Boyden The Impact of Civilization on the Biology of Man. University of Toronto Press, 1970: 48-68.

Fenner calculated that 3000 cases are required in a year to maintain measles, and this would need a population of about 300,000.[19] On the basis of American experience Cockburn suggested that a population of 1,000,000 is near the threshold required to establish measles as a recurrent epidemic infection.[20] Perhaps the most satisfactory data were provided by Black (see table 2.1), who showed that in island populations below 500,000 measles disappeared unless reintroduced.[21] The general conclusion drawn from such evidence is that most human infections could not have been established until the populations in frequent contact reached many thousands.

[18] Hamer, W. H. 'Epidemic diseases in England.' *Lancet*, 1906: 735.

[19] Fenner, F. 'Infectious disease and social change.' *Med. J. Australia*, 1971, 1: 1043, 1099.

[20] Cockburn, A. Where did our infectious diseases come from?

[21] Black, F. L. 'Measles endemnicity in insular populations: critical community size and its evolutionary implications' *J. Theoret. Biol.* 1966, II: 207–11.

The great change in community size is believed to have begun about 6000 years ago (see table 2.2); before that time human settlements consisted of villages with less than 300 persons, much too small to maintain the human infections. It was only after the introduction of improved farming techniques, particularly irrigated agriculture, that a few cities had 100,000 persons, and only in the last few centuries after industrialization that they had half a million. Remarkably, we owe the origin of most serious infectious diseases to the conditions which led to our cultural heritage, the city states made possible by the planting of crops in the flood plains of Mesopotamia, Egypt and the Indus Valley.

Table 2.2 The time scale of cultural changes in man, in relation to the number of generations and the size of human communities

Years before 1968	Generations	Cultural state	Size of human communities
1,000,000	50,000	hunter and foodgatherer	scattered nomadic bands of <100 persons
10,000	500	development of agriculture	relatively settled villages of <300 persons
5,500	220	development of irrigated agriculture	few cities of 100,000; mostly villages of <300 persons
250	10	introduction of steam power	some cities of 500,000, many cities of 100,000; many villages of 1,000 persons
130	5	introduction of sanitary reforms	

Source: Fenner, 'The effects of changing social organization on the infectious diseases of man.

Defective hygiene The conditions which resulted from agriculture had a profound effect on the frequency of exposure to infectious disease. The most important influence was the proximity of large numbers of people, which facilitated the spread of airborne and other infections. But hygienic conditions were also significant, particulary those determined by methods of handling food and water and disposing of excreta and waste. Cholera, as we have noted (see p. 38), appeared when villages and village water supplies were established, and malaria became serious when 'the size of human populations and the opportunities for breeding of vectors increased with advances in agricultural practices.'[22] Tuberculosis, possibly an ancient disease, could almost be described as a disease of cities, for it became a common cause of death under the conditions prevailing in large

[22] Fenner, F. The effects of changing social organisation on the diseases of man.

towns. The spread of intestinal infections – typhoid, dysentery, tuberculosis, salmonella and the like – resulted from contamination of food and water. So the hygienic conditions which followed the introduction of agriculture made it possible for new diseases to appear, and for some diseases already present to become more serious.

Insufficient food The third of the major influences on the infections is, remarkably, the most controversial. For most people who have worked with sick children in developing countries, it seems unquestionable that malnutrition has a profound effect on the frequency and seriousness of infectious diseases, and the World Health Organization referred to an adequate diet as the most effective 'vaccine' against most diarrhoeal, respiratory and other common infections. Yet this conclusion has been questioned by demographers who are unimpressed by the clinical and experimental findings. The issue is so important in the history of health that it will be worthwhile to consider briefly some of the difficulties which beset the search for conclusive evidence.

First, there are obvious problems in conducting experiments on infectious diseases in laboratory animals. It is difficult to find a species which can be infected in sufficient numbers with a particular organism, and to observe the effects of varying the diet under controlled conditions. It is not surprising that laboratory evidence is inconclusive, and that we rely more on observations on man himself and wild animals.

A second problem arises because malnutrition occurs chiefly among the poor, and it is often difficult to separate the effects of food shortage from those of other features of poverty. For example, populations in which tuberculosis, or, in a tropical country, schistosomiasis, are common are likely to be both underfed and heavily exposed to infection, and it is not easy to distinguish between the effects of the two influences.

A further problem is that the malnutrition common in developing countries today, and in all countries in the recent past, is not necessarily, indeed is not usually, of an easily recognizable type, such as rickets, beriberi, pellagra or the protein calorie deficiency syndromes, kwaskiorkor and marasmus. As already noted (see p. 46) it occurs most often as chronic malnutrition without specific features.

Another difficulty is that the effects of malnutrition are not the same in all infectious diseases: they are marked in diarrhoea, measles and tuberculosis, but less obvious in whooping cough and malaria.

Finally, we all know from personal experience that good nutrition may not prevent the occurrence of infectious disease. All social classes are susceptible to the common respiratory and intestinal infections, and in the past serious diseases such as smallpox, plague and tuberculosis infected and killed both well-to-do and poor people.

In spite of the difficulties, it is evident that the state of health of an individual has a considerable bearing on response to infection. Measles is a conspicuous example of a condition in which infection rates are high in all social classes, but the likelihood of serious illness and death depends largely on the health of the child and is much increased in the poor. It is also clear that the general state of health is largely influenced by previous illnesses and malnutrition.

It is more difficult to go beyond these generalizations to a precise estimate of the part played by nutrition in determining the frequency and outcome of infection. There are many conflicting reports in the literature, and in the past, disorders of metabolism and food deficiency were accorded a relatively minor role in relation to the health of man and other animals. However, these views have changed and Newberne and Williams have summarized recent thinking.[23] 'The ultimate effect of an infection depends to a considerable degree on the nutritional adequacy of the animal at the time of exposure to the agent. A severe degree of deficiency of almost any of the essential nutrients may have a marked effect on the manner in which the host responds to the effect of an infectious agent. Abundant evidence clearly indicates that the same infection may be mild or even unapparent in a well nourished animal, but virulent and sometimes fatal in one that is malnourished.' They referred to four ways in which malnutrition influences infection: '(1) by effects on the host which facilitate initial invasion of the infectious agent; (2) through an effect on the agent once it is established on the tissues; (3) through an effect on secondary infection; or (4) by retarding convalescence from infection.' They concluded that:

grossly inadequate intakes of protein and other specific nutrients are today resulting in extreme degrees of malnutrition and concomitant infectious disease. It seems likely that the interaction between nutrition and infection is more important in animal and human populations than one would predict from the results of laboratory investigations. It must be remembered that the interaction between nutrition and infection is dynamic, being frequently characterized by synergism and, less commonly, by antagonism, and that the control of malnutrition and infection are interdependent, so that the course of a disease is intimately related to the nutritional status of the host.

Knowledge of the relation between malnutrition and infection in man has been extended considerably by the experience of the World Health Organization in developing countries where infectious diseases are still rampant. The experience leaves no doubt that malnutrition contributes largely to the high level of infectious deaths; ill fed populations are more

[23] Newberne, P. M. and Williams, G. 'Nutritional influences on the course of infections.' In: Dunlop, R. H. and Moon, H. W. *Resistance to Infectious Disease.* Saskatoon, Modern Press, 1970: 93.

prone to infections and suffer more seriously when they are infected.[24] Moreover, infectious diseases have an unfavourable effect on nutritional state, and the interaction between disease and malnutrition leads to a vicious cycle which is characteristic of poverty and underdevelopment. The effects are not restricted to respiratory and intestinal infections for which there are no specific vaccines; mortality is high from measles and whooping cough for which effective vaccination is available. The problems are particularly serious in infancy, before the child has developed its own defence mechanisms. The World Health Organization concluded that 'one half to three quarters of all statistically recorded deaths of infants and young children are attributed to a combination of malnutrition and infection'.[25] The deficiency is due mainly to lack of calories and proteins, although mineral and vitamin deficiencies are often associated.

A debilitated organism is far less resistant to attacks by invading micro-organisms. Ordinary measles or diarrhoea – harmless and short-lived diseases among well fed children – are usually serious and often fatal to the chronically malnourished. Before vaccines existed, practically every child in all countries caught measles, but 300 times more deaths occurred in the poorer countries than in the richer ones. The reason was not that the virus was more virulent, nor that there were fewer medical services; but that in poorly nourished communities the microbes attack a host which, because of chronic malnutrition, is less able to resist. The same happens with diarrhoea, respiratory infections, tuberculosis and many other common infections to which malnourished populations pay a heavy and unnecessary toll.[26]

The report gave the results of a recent investigation of mortality in infancy in Latin America, which concluded that 'when malnutrition was not given as the major cause of death in official statistics, it was an associated cause in 57 per cent of all deaths among children under five and, in some regions, in two thirds of these deaths. Diarrhoeal infections accounted for most of the deaths, with malnutrition as an associated cause in 50–80 per cent of the deaths attributable to measles'. The author concluded that malnutrition was the most serious health problem in the populations studied.

   These and other investigations show the enormous importance of nutrition in determining the outcome of infection. The World Health Organization report suggested that 'we have given too much attention to the enemy and have to some extent overlooked our own defences'; that is to say we have concentrated on specific measures such as vaccination and treatment without sufficient regard for the predominant part played by nutritional state.

[24] Scrimshaw, N. W., Taylor, C. E. and Gordon, J. E. *Interaction of Nutrition and Infection.* Geneva, World Health Organization 1968.

[25] World Health Organization. 'Better food for a healthier world.' *Features* FS / **19**, 1973.

[26] Behar, M. 'A deadly combination.' *World Health*, February-March, 1974: 29.

Although historical evidence is inevitably incomplete, there is little doubt that in the past malnutrition and infectious diseases were frequently associated. Braudel regarded it as a commonplace that famine opens the door to epidemics, and he referred to the close link between the dates of famines and epidemics in eighteenth-century Mexico. He concluded that 'undernourishment, on all the evidence, is a "multiplying" factor in the spread of diseases', and quoted appreciatively the Tuscan proverb: 'The best remedy against malaria is a well filled pot.'[27]

Although the importance of the well-filled pot is now widely accepted, doubts are sometimes expressed about its value in diseases such as plague, influenza and malaria, on the grounds that the rich as well as the poor are affected. Nevertheless there are class differences in experience of these diseases, determined partly by different frequencies of exposure but also by the better nutrition of the well-to-do. It is probably true to say that response to any infectious disease depends on the state of health of the individual, and the state of health is influenced powerfully by nutrition.

Sources of human infections Although knowledge of infectious diseases in the wild is still very incomplete, it is now clear that many human parasites had precursors in other animals. This subject has been discussed extensively by Cockburn, who quoted the remark that 'like hosts have like parasites', and cited several examples – intestinal protozoa, worms, malaria parasites, the scabies mite, herpes virus, infective hepatitis virus and possibly syphilis and treponematoses. There has been a continuous exchange of infective organisms between man and other animals, the outcome of the exchange being determined by climatic, social and other conditions.[28] Contact with other animals increased under agriculture, with domesticated animals such as cattle, sheep, goats, pigs, horses, cats and dogs, and with unwanted intruders attracted to human settlements, such as rats, mice, sparrows, ticks, fleas and mosquitos.

Many micro-organisms are host specific, and most of the countless invaders with which man was brought into contact would not successfully infect him. Occasionally, however, one would succeed, and if it could be transferred from man to man the stage would be set for establishment of a human pathogen.[29]

Fenner[30] and Fiennes[31] have discussed the sources of human infections and the animals from which diseases were probably acquired. Measles, for

27 Braudel, F. *Structure of Everyday Life*: 81.
28 Cockburn, A. Where did our infectious diseases come from?
29 *Ibid.*
30 Fenner, F. Effects of changing social organization on the diseases of man.
31 Fiennes, R. N. *Zoonoses and the Origins and Ecology of Human Disease*. London, Academic Press, 1978: 35.

example, is believed to have come from dogs, since the measles virus is closely related to the viruses of canine distemper and rinderpest. The many rhinoviruses which cause the common cold appear to be derived from horses which are the only natural hosts. The human type of the tubercle bacillus which causes respiratory tuberculosis probably resulted from mutation by the bovine type, which was transferred to man from wild cattle. Fiennes suggested that the water buffalo is possibly the original source of leprosy, the cow of diphtheria and the monkey of syphilis. Many other diseases such as mumps and smallpox are believed to have arisen from related conditions in other animals, although the original hosts are not certainly known. Fiennes also reviewed the origins of the few diseases which are capable of spreading as global pandemics. In order to do this they must: 'be capable of rapid transmission from one host to another'; 'find susceptible hosts in sufficient numbers to maintain the momentum'; and (to fulfil the first criterion) 'must be spread by airborne infection'. Only two diseases – plague and influenza – have met these exacting require-ments. Plague is believed to have originated as an inapparent infection of gerbils in eastern Asia, and the first great pandemic occurred in the years AD 592-594. The human virus of influenza appears to be identified with the virus of swine influenza, and it is thought that new pandemic strains of influenza A viruses arise as zoonoses.

As we shall consider later the decline of infectious diseases from the eighteenth century, it is important to be clear about the reasons for their earlier predominance. The large and aggregated populations of cities made it possible for the human infections to exist, and high exposure and low resistance made them predominant during most of the historical period. The high exposure was due partly to defective hygiene (see p. 51). As subsequent experience has shown, even in crowded cities a population can protect itself against some infections by hygienic measures.

But the impact of the diseases was greatly increased by low resistance, determined by ill health, poor nutrition and stress. There is good evidence that stress is an important influence in respiratory infections,[32] and it is quite likely that it has an effect in many, perhaps most, infectious diseases. However it is not possible to assess the extent of stress at different periods of history, although some people have attempted to do so, often under the questionable conviction that stress has greatly increased in modern life. As most of our predecessors lived short lives in or near to poverty, it is probable that life has always been stressful, and for influences that lowered resistance to the human infections in the agricultural period we must look mainly to the related problems of ill health and malnutrition.

[32] Totman, R., Reed, S. E. and Craig, J. W. 'Cognitive dissonance stress and virus-induced common colds.' *J. Psychosom. Res.* 1977, **21**: 55–63.

Population-Growth

If a generalization may be risked about the rate of population growth in the agricultural period, it is that it was much faster than the rate that preceded it and much slower than the one that followed. Since the population of the world is unknown before the eighteenth century and is not accurately recorded for the present day, these conclusions may be questioned. But the estimates that have been made suggest that 10,000 years ago the total was below, and probably well below, 10 million; in 1800 it was almost 1000 million and it has now reached 5000 million. Even allowing for gross inaccuracy of these figures, there is little doubt that numbers increased more rapidly in the few thousand years that followed the agricultural revolution than in the few million that preceded it. Yet the rate was slow when compared with that which has prevailed in the last few centuries.

One other general point should be made. In the period when some estimates can be accepted without serious reservations – say between the fifteenth and eighteenth centuries – the rate of growth varied widely at different times. This variation is concealed in the crude estimates of the long-term trend of world population. There are, therefore, two major questions to be considered in relation to population growth in the agricultural period. Why was the rate of growth faster than in the hunter gatherer period? How can we account for the rapid increase at certain times and places?

Among the most courageous estimates of early world population are those of McEvedy and Jones,[33] who divided the time since 10,000 BC with three cycles, primary, medieval and modern. They suggested that the population increased quite slowly in the first half of the primary cycle, from about 4 million in 10,000 BC to 5 million in 5000 BC. From that time numbers rose rapidly, and reached 100 million in 500 BC and nearly 200 million by the second century AD. The rate of growth then began to decline: 'The gain over the period 500 BC to AD 1 was 70% not 100%: over the next 200 years the addition was a mere 12% and then growth ceased entirely. The cycle that had begun 6,000 years earlier . . . was complete.'

In the medieval period numbers are said to have increased again, from about 190 million in AD 500 to 350 million in AD 1400. The modern rise of population (with which we shall be concerned later) may be taken to have started in the eighteenth century, when the population was about 750 million (in 1750). It rose to 2000 million in 1930 and to 4000 million in 1975.

[33] McEvedy, C. and Jones, R. *Atlas of World Population*. London, Penguin, 1985.

With due regard for the unreliability of most of these estimates, we can accept that the population of the world expanded only slowly for several thousand years after the agricultural revolution; that it began to rise from about 5000 BC; and that a much more rapid rate of increase appeared in, or just before, the eighteenth century.

While crude estimates of world population are perhaps sufficient to indicate long-term trends, they conceal the variation in growth rates in different places. The variation may have occurred on a limited scale in the millenia after the agricultural revolution, but when discussing the populations of single countries we are restricted to recent periods. Even then, there is little reliable evidence before the nineteenth century: almost nothing is known about non-Chinese Asia outside Japan, about India, about Oceania or about Africa south of the Sahara.[34] The most useful estimates are for Europe and China.

In Western Europe there were prolonged increases of population between 1100 and 1350, and between 1450 and 1650. In China from 1683 there was a century of rapid growth, when numbers rose from about 150 million (in 1700) to 313 million (in 1774).[35] However, the periods of rapid growth were not confined to these areas. Indeed, Braudel concluded that long-term fluctuations occurred 'more or less simultaneously from one end of the inhabited world to the other: 'China and India probably advanced and regressed in the same rhythm as the West'. He suggested that 'the synchronism is evident in the eighteenth century and is more than probable in the nineteenth. It can be assumed that it also applied to the thirteenth and stretched from the France of St. Louis to the remote China of the Mongols.'[36]

How are we to account for the increase in rates of population growth, and for its remarkable occurrence at about the same time in countries which differed widely in economic, social and climatic conditions? The primary influences are food and disease, and we need to assess the relation between the two.

Throughout the agricultural period, rates of population growth were determined largely by the availability of food. Before the nineteenth century most people were chronically undernourished, and exposed at intervals to the devastating effects of famine. France, a relatively privileged country, is said to have had '10 *general* famines during the tenth century, 26 in the eleventh, 2 in the twelfth, 4 in the fourteenth, 7 in the fifteenth, 13 in the sixteenth, 11 in the seventeenth and 16 in the eighteenth.' Conditions were at least as bad in other countries of Europe and much worse in Asia.[37]

---

[34] Braudel, F. 1985, *op. cit.*: 31–51.
[35] McNeill, W. H. *Plagues and Peoples.*
[36] Braudel, F. *Structure of Everyday Life.*
[37] *Ibid.*

The last major famines occurred in England in the 1620s, in Scotland in the 1690s, in Germany, Switzerland and Scandinavia in 1732, in France in 1795 and in Ireland, with the failure of the potato crop, in the 1840s.[38]

It is an indication of the importance of food that an increase in supplies usually coincided with a sustained expansion of numbers. In China the growth of population after 1683 was accompanied by an agricultural revolution based on new crops, improved agricultural methods, and the use of additional land both within and outside the country. In Europe in the eighteenth and nineteenth centuries there was a great advance in food production, in Britain sufficient to feed a population which trebled between 1700 and 1850 with little supplement from imported foods. 'A correlation obviously exists between the rise in yields and the rise in population.'[39]

I have already referred to the importance of infectious diseases; as the predominant causes of death they inevitably had a large influence on population growth. The history of the great pandemic infections has been extensively recorded, but there were many other diseases – typhus, syphilis, smallpox and the like – which also had devastating effects on mortality and population growth, more localized and for shorter periods.

When assessing the two primary influences – food and disease – we are again brought back to the question of the relation between the two. Probably no-one doubts that both were important: without more food the populations of China and Europe could not have expanded; and at many times disease played a large part in limiting population growth. In his review of the influence of infectious diseases in history McNeill concluded that: 'Changes in disease patterns and the increase in productivity that the spread of American food crops permitted were probably the two most active factors in triggering civilized population growth in early modern times. They operated world-wide, and in parallel fashion to allow more human beings to survive and grow to maturity than had ever been possible before'.[40]

Moreover, it is well recognized that the two influences are closely related. In his general examination of demographic changes between the fifteenth and eighteenth centuries Braudel stated: 'A balance between mouths to be fed and the difficulties of feeding them, between manpower and jobs, is re-established by epidemics and famines (the second preceding or accompanying the first).'[41] The point is well illustrated by experience of the Black Death, which was preceded by serious food shortages that spread throughout Europe betwen 1308 and 1318. 'Famine was never an isolated event. Sooner or later it opened the door to epidemics.'[42]

[38] Grigg, D. The World Food Problem. Oxford, Basil Blackwell, 1985: 33.
[39] Braudel, F. Structure of Everyday Life: 123.
[40] McNeill, W. H. Plagues and Peoples.
[41] Braudel, F. Structures of Everyday Life.
[42] Ibid.

In spite of these generalizations, doubts are still expressed about the relation between food and infectious disease. Historians have concluded 'that every pathogenic agent has its own history, which runs parallel to that of its victims, and that the evolution of the diseases largely depends on changes, and sometimes mutations, in the agents themselves. Here lies the cause of the complicated advances and retreats of disease, the surprise appearances of epidemic outbreaks, and the quiescence and sometimes complete disappearance of certain illnesses.'[43] According to this view a considerable part of the history of infectious diseases cannot be accounted for by nutritional or other environmental causes, and must be attributed to genetic changes in micro-organisms.

Perhaps the first thing that should be said about this appraisal is that up to a point it is credible. Probably some major epidemics of the past were not due predominantly to malnutrition, although it is likely that all were made worse by it. But historians have tended to overestimate the effects of the occasional killing diseases, and the epidemic infections have been accorded a disproportionate place in the history of infectious disease. Even Braudel, the indefatigable historian, confessed himself defeated by the 'over-plentiful documentation' of plague. The death rate from plague was estimated as between 40 and 60 per cent,[44] and the influenza pandemic of 1918–19 is said to have killed between 15 and 25 million people in all countries. But even if these estimates are accepted – and in periods of such high mortality they are likely to have included many deaths from other causes – the effects on long-term trends were limited. For it must be remembered that until the eighteenth century about seven out of every ten people born were dead before maturity, mainly from endemic causes of infant and child mortality, such as gastroenteritis, pneumonia and malnutrition. To explain the slow rates of population growth we have chiefly to account for the high level of these deaths in every year, rather than for the heavy mortality from epidemic infections in exceptional years.

The two main determinants were the frequency of exposure and the extent of the body's resistance to infectious diseases. As we have seen, exposure to infection was greatly increased by crowding and poor hygiene; and malnutrition was the chief reason for low resistance. One of the most important conclusions that will be drawn from examination of the modern rise of population (chapter 3) is that in the nineteenth century improvement in nutrition led to a large reduction of infectious deaths, even when exposure to infection substantially increased.

In the light of this conclusion we can now consider a general interpretation of the major changes in the world population during the agricultural

43 *Ibid.*
44 *Ibid.*

period. Until about 5000 BC population growth was slow because the area under cultivation was too small, and methods of production too primitive, to make it possible to feed large numbers. From that time improved farming methods, particularly the use of irrigation in river deltas, made it possible for numbers to rise, and they increased to the size which allowed the human infectious diseases to become established. But as population growth was not effectively restricted by control of fertility or deliberate killing, numbers expanded to the size at which food supplies became again marginal. Food shortage was reinstated as the major cause of sickness and death, but with this difference from the period of hunting and gathering, that its effects were manifested largely through experience of infectious disease. It was the infections which caused the high death rates, but it was malnutrition which largely determined the occurrence and outcome of most infections.

The same explanation can be given for the remarkable growth of population in different countries at about the same time: it was due essentially to increased food production which led to a reduction of mortality. The question remains as to the reasons for widespread improvement in agricultural productivity, and it is possible that it was due largely to climatic changes, as Braudel suggested.[45] But if so they were a secondary rather than a primary influence, and the main determinant of the rate of population growth was food.

Stating this interpretation, one is aware of the risk of being thought to overstate it. I should therefore stress that it does not overlook the importance of exposure to infection, or the changing character of infectious diseases, or the profound short term effects of pandemic infections such as influenza and plague. The interpretation is based on two conclusions which are often overlooked: that the most important influences on mortality were not the occasional dramatic epidemic infections, but the endemic causes of death which killed most people; and that the level of endemic deaths was determined essentially by population size and the availability of food.

In summary: The knowledge needed for agriculture is believed to have been available long before it was applied. But hunting and gathering was a successful form of life, and it was abandoned only when food requirements could no longer be met in the traditional ways, by reducing demands through limiting numbers and by increasing supplies through acceptance of different foods or occupation of new territories. There was a reciprocal relation between food technology and population growth. The demands of a (slowly) rising population led to adoption of agriculture, but it was the food provided by agriculture that made possible the subsequent increase of numbers.

[45] *Ibid.*

In relation to health the most significant consequences of the change to agriculture were the expansion of populations and the creation of densely populated and unhygienic urban areas. The pattern of non-communicable diseases was not altered substantially by those developments; diseases such as cancer, heart disease and diabetes were still rare, although the replacement of a varied plant and animal diet by one based on a few cereals opened the way to some vitamin and protein deficiencies. But experience of infectious diseases was transformed about 5000 years ago by the rapid growth of population and the establishment of cities. They provided ideal conditions for the human infections, diseases caused by organisms which have no other animal host and require large numbers of people in close contact for their propagation and spread. Most of these infections could not have existed in hunter-gatherers, as they were acquired from domesticated and other animals. Infectious diseases became the predominant causes of sickness and death; and the endemic ones, constantly present, had a much greater effect than the occasional epidemic infections (such as plague) which had devastating effects for short periods.

The predominance of infectious diseases was due essentially to the combined effects of high exposure and low resistance to infection caused mainly by poor nutrition. Thus the causes of sickness and death under agriculture resembled those of the hunting and gathering period in that food deficiency was still critical, but differed in that its effects were manifested largely through experience of infectious disease.

The additional food provided by agriculture made it possible for numbers to increase; but the increase was not effectively limited by social restraints (control of fertility and deliberate killing), and populations expanded to the size at which food supplies became again marginal. Famine was common, and the relatively slow rate of population growth was due essentially to defective hygiene and food deficiency.

3

Industry

As we have seen, the transition to agriculture from hunting and gathering, the first of the two major changes in conditions of human life, occurred in a period of a few thousand years. By leading to the predominance of infectious diseases as causes of sickness and death, it had a large effect on health and a considerable effect on population growth. The second change, to industry, is taking place in a much shorter period, at most a few hundred years. Its effects on health and population growth are even more profound, chiefly as a result of the decline of the infections and their replacement by non-communicable diseases. In this Chapter I shall try to unravel the multiple influences which have led to these events.

The Modern Rise of Population

The increase of numbers which began at about the end of the seventeenth century and has continued to the present day will be referred to as the modern rise of population. When cultivation of plants and domestication of animals began, the population of the world was below 10 million: by 1830 it has increased to 1000 million; it was 2000 million in 1930, 3000 in 1960, 4000 in 1975 and 5000 in 1987 (see figure 3.1). That is to say, it took hundreds of thousands of years for the human population to expand to the first thousand million, the second was added in 100 years, the third in 30, the fourth in 15 and the fifth in 12.

The growth of the population of England and Wales was even more remarkable. It is shown in figure 3.2, from the eleventh century, when it was estimated as one and a half million by a count of families for the Domesday Book. The population increased to five and a half million in 1700, 18 in 1851 and 49 in 1971. For investigation of population growth, English data have two advantages, the modern increase appears to have begun somewhat earlier than in other countries, and cause of death was recorded nationally on death certificates from 1838. Elsewhere this information is not available before the late nineteenth century.

It is important to decide at the outset whether the modern rise is to be regarded as analogous to earlier increases of population, given particular but not unique significance because of its coincidence with industrialization. If so, it seems permissible to argue by analogy and to invoke the same kinds of explanations as are proposed for earlier periods. This treatment has indeed been adopted by some demographers, who attribute the eighteenth century increase to a decline of mortality brought about by fortuitous changes in the behaviour of infectious diseases, or even of a single disease such as plague. But if the modern increase was essentially different from earlier ones, so too are likely to be the reasons for it.

The modern rise is distinguished from all previous increases by its size, its continuity and its duration. The scale of the changes shown in figures 3.1 and 3.2 leaves no doubt that we are dealing with a unique phenomenon; but also, unlike any previous rise, it has continued for nearly three centuries, and a major challenge of our times is to bring it to an end.

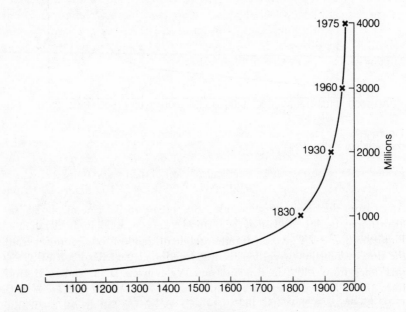

Figure 3.1 The modern rise of world population
Source: The Modern Rise of Population: 2

In Britain the increase probably began in the eighteenth century. It was well advanced before births and deaths were registered, and even by the time of the first census in 1801, the rate of increase was much greater than any that preceded it. For the purpose of interpreting the modern rise of population it is unnecessary, and probably impossible, to judge precisely when it started. It is sufficient to know that whatever the trend in the early years of the eighteenth century, at some time well before its close the unique expansion had begun.

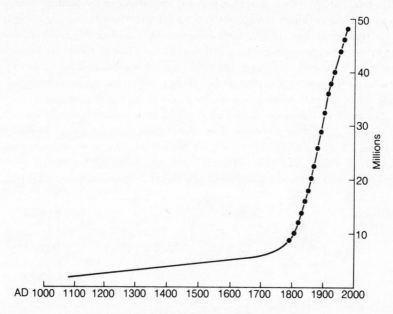

Figure 3.2 The modern rise of population in England and Wales
Source: as figure 3.1.

Fertility and Mortality

Apart from the effects of migration, an increase in the rate of population growth may be due to a rise of the birth rate and, or, a fall in the death rate. Figures 3.3 and 3.4 give birth rates and death rates of four countries from the times when they were first recorded nationally: in Sweden from 1749; in France from 1800; in England and Wales from 1838; and in Ireland from 1871. They provide no evidence that the rates have increased.

In England and Wales the birth rate began to fall in 1871–80; the increase during the period 1841–50 is usually attributed to deficient registration in the early years. The death rate was fairly constant for the two decades after registration, but fell from 1861–70.

The Swedish data are of particular interest, since they are available from 1751. During the second half of the eighteenth century the birth rate and

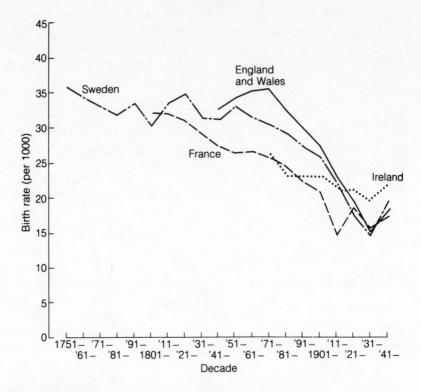

Figure 3.3 Birth rates from the times when first registered
Source: as figure 3.1: 28.

death rate were high and fluctuating, the birth rate being generally above 30 (per 1000 population), and the death rate above 25, rates similar to those estimated for England and Wales in the same period. The death rate began to fall during the early nineteenth century, while the birth rate continued at about the eighteenth century level until the third quarter, when it also declined.

The contributions of the birth rate and death rate to the early growth of the Swedish population can be estimated as follows. The population increased by 28 per cent between 1761-5 and 1801-10 and by 54 per cent between 1811-15 and 1856-60. For the two fifty year periods mean birth rates were the same (32.6), and mean death rates were 27.6 and 22.7 respectively. Thus the increase of population between 1750 and 1850 was clearly due to a reduction of mortality; the increase during the second half of the eighteenth century, when mortality remained more or less constant, is attributable to the continuing difference between births and deaths

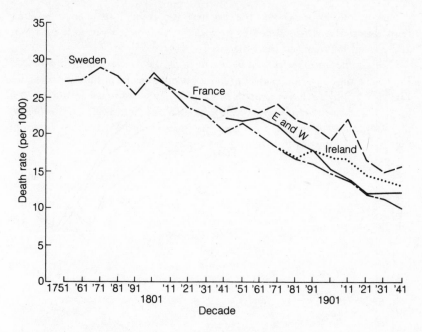

Figure 3.4 Death rates from the times when first registered
Source: as figure 3.3.

established by the middle of the century. For the whole period, 1751–1800, the birth rate was 33.6 per 1000 and the death rate 27.4.

In France, the death rate fell from 1800 until the middle of the century; it then remained fairly constant until about 1875 when it again declined. The rate in France (24) was somewhat higher than in England and Wales (22) in 1850. However, the most remarkable difference between the two countries was in the behaviour of the birth rate, which fell in France almost continuously from 1800, at least seventy years earlier than in England and Wales. At the middle of the nineteenth century, the birth rates in France and in England and Wales were 27 and 34 respectively.

In Ireland, because of deficiencies of data, no confident conclusions can be drawn about the rates before 1871, except that a considerable excess of births over deaths had been established by that time. There was a reduction of the birth rate during the last three decades of the nineteenth century, when the death rate was more or less constant. However, a substantial excess of births over deaths remained, and indeed throughout the period 1871–1950 the decline of the birth rate and the decline of the death rate were remarkably similar.

Considered as a whole, the records for these four countries since registration of births and deaths provide no evidence of rising birth rates, and indeed for much of the time the rates were falling.

One of the most remarkable features of the demographic history of Europe is the variation between countries in rates of population growth. Figure 3.5 shows relative growth rates in the four countries between 1700, for which the estimated populations are taken as 1, and 1950. In this period the population increased 8.0 times in England and Wales, 5.3 times in Sweden, 2.0 times in France and 1.7 times in Ireland.

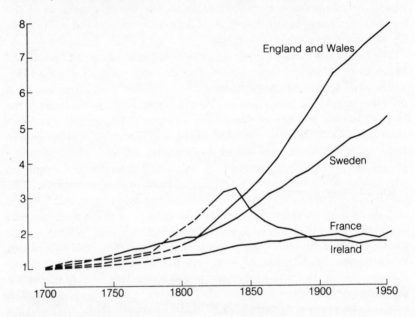

Figure 3.5 Sizes of populations relative to their sizes in 1700
Source: as figure 3.1: 32.

When assessing the reasons for these differences it is essential to consider the effects of migration. They can be estimated by comparing the actual rates of population growth with those that would have resulted if population size were determined only by the prevailing birth and death rates with no losses or additions from migration.[1] The estimates can of course be made only from the time when births and deaths were first recorded: 1841 when Sweden and France are compared with England and Wales, and 1871 in the case of Ireland. These data are relatively late in the history of the

[1] McKeown, T., Record, R. G. and Brown, R. G. 'An interpretation of the modern rise of population in Europe.' *Population Studies*, 1972, **27**: 345.

modern rise of population, but they include the periods when emigration was at its height.

In Sweden, from 1841, elimination of the effects of migration substantially increases the estimate of population, whereas in England and Wales there is only a small difference between the calculated and actual numbers. Indeed the calculated rates of population growth are very similar in Sweden and England and Wales, so that the difference between the actual rates in this period was determined almost entirely by emigration from Sweden. However, this was not considerable before 1860, so that some other explanation must be sought for the slower expansion of the Swedish population before that time. It is probably to be found in the lower Swedish birth rate.

The rate of population growth was slower in France than in England and Wales from 1800, and the two rates had diverged considerably by 1841, when birth and death rates became available for both countries. It is therefore possible to investigate the effects of migration on only part of the large difference in rates of population increase which occurred between 1800 and 1950. The slower growth of the population of France between 1841 and 1951 is not explained by emigration. Indeed, throughout the period the increase was greater for the actual than for the calculated population, which indicates that migration resulted in a net increase. The explanation for the difference in growth rates between France and England and Wales must therefore be sought in the behaviour of the birth rate and death rate. Both contributed to the difference. From 1841 to 1950, except for a short time, the birth rate was lower in France than in England and Wales and the death rate was considerably higher. Over most of the period the influence of the lower birth rate was somewhat greater than that of the higher death rate.

Although it is not possible to assess the effect of emigration from Ireland by the method described above before 1871, when births and deaths were first registered, its earlier influence on population size is evident. The population of Ireland was increasing at about the same rate as that of England and Wales during most of the first half of the nineteenth century. Large scale emigration began in the fifth decade, and from that time the population fell sharply. Comparison between the actual rate of population growth in Ireland from 1871 to 1950 and the rate which would have resulted if population size had been determined solely by the numbers of births and deaths, shows that emigration was the main, although not the only reason for the difference between growth rates in Ireland and England and Wales.

The contributions of birth and death rates to the difference can also be estimated. From 1871 to 1911 approximately, the birth rate was considerably higher in England and Wales than in Ireland, and this was the main reason for the residual difference in rates of population growth over that period, not accounted for by emigration from Ireland. From 1931 the birth rate was lower in England and Wales, and from this time until 1950 the rate of increase of the calculated population was a little greater in Ireland. The contribution of death rate differences over the whole period from 1871 to 1950 was relatively small.

We can now summarize conclusions concerning the contribution of births and deaths to the growth of population since the rates were registered nationally. In the four countries considered, the rise of population was due to an excess of births over deaths established by the time of registration, and to a subsequent fall of mortality. The slower rates of population growth in the other three countries than in England and Wales are attributable mainly to emigration, in the case of Ireland and Sweden, and to a lower birth rate in the case of France. At least from the time of registration, it is the decline of mortality that has to be explained in order to account for the rapid expansion of population.

However, this conclusion has been said to overlook recent work on pre-industrial populations, which indicates that the decline of mortality accelerated rather than initiated population growth. In the most extensive investigation that has been made, data from parish registers were used to provide estimates of population growth, fertility, nuptiality and mortality in England and Wales from the sixteenth to the nineteenth century.[2] This work is said to show that changes in fertility rather than in mortality were the major influences on the modern rise of population. It should be noted that what is in question is not whether fertility was at times reduced – undoubtedly it was – but whether in the modern period it was the main influence.

When considering the evidence from parish registers it is essential to recognize their limitations. The registers record baptisms, marriages and burials, and too few records now exist to provide an accurate national picture. National estimates of population during the eighteenth century are based on replies to a question in the 1801 census, asking for the number of baptisms and burials in each 'Parish, Township or Place' for each decadal year from 1700 to 1780 and for every year from then until 1800. Thus, for the greater part of the eighteenth century there are figures only for every tenth year, some of which are recognized to be exceptional demographically.

Even at the time of the census, however, the registers on which the returns were based were known to be incomplete, and to obtain national

[2] Wrigley, E. A. and Schofield, R. *The Population History of England. 541-1871: A Reconstruction*. Cambridge, Massachusetts Harvard University Press 1981.

estimates, allowance had to be made for unregistered births and deaths. 'The estimates for birth and death rates are highly sensitive to the allowances that the particular estimator sees fit to make, and the evidence on this point is so scanty that we do not know within a very wide margin what the right allowance would be.'[3] For the period prior to the Marriage Act of 1753 'it is impossible to make a valid statement about the rate of marriage from the study of a single parish' and 'the difficulties in calculating the rate of birth to which the marriages give rise is even greater'.[4]

To complicate matters further, the accuracy of individual registers varied from year to year. After a review of parish sources Krause concluded that 'parochial registration was relatively accurate in the early eighteenth century, became somewhat less so in the 1780's, virtually collapsed between roughly 1795 and 1820 and then improved somewhat between 1821 and 1837'.[5] However, even this appraisal must be viewed with caution: a report of 1774 on the population of Manchester stated that 'this account does not include the deaths or births, amongst the Dissenters. These, by a late improvement in our bills of mortality, are now admitted into the parish register.'[6] How late the improvement was we are not told, but on figures averaged over the previous five years it has the effect of raising the number of deaths by nearly 6 per cent, and of births by over 18 per cent. Presumably at some earlier period Dissenters were not included, although how much earlier, and whether they contributed proportionately in the same way to births and deaths, is unknown.

It is indeed difficult to judge the reliability of the registers at any time during the eighteenth century. The allowances needed for under-registration must have varied from place to place and from year to year, and are still in dispute. But in any case, the variation in fertility and mortality from one area to another makes it unlikely that an acceptable national picture could emerge from an analysis of individual registers.

The conclusion drawn from work on parish registers – that the decline of mortality accelerated rather than initiated population growth – implies (a) that the growth of population was due initially to a rise in the birth rate brought about by withdrawal of restraints on fertility, and (b) that a change in mortality was a later and, overall, less significant influence. In relation to

[3] Habbakuk, H. J. 'The economic history of modern Britain.' In: Glass, D. V. and Eversley, D. E. C. (eds) *Population in History*, London, Edward Arnold, 1965: 149.

[4] Chambers, J. D. *Population, Economy and Society in Pre-Industrial Britain*. London, Oxford University Press, 1972: 59.

[5] Krause, J. T. 'The changing adequacy of English registration, 1600–1837.' In: *Population in History, op. cit.*: 393.

[6] Percival, T. 'Observations on the state of population in Manchester.' *Philosophical Transactions of the Royal Society*, 1774, **64**.

the changes of the last three centuries the latter is the more important issue and will be considered first.

As the birth rate and death rate in England and Wales were much higher in the eighteenth century than they are today, and since the birth rate has been falling for most of the time since it was recorded, it would seem almost self-evident that the decline of mortality was the more important influence on population growth. However, as this conclusion has been questioned, it will be necessary to support it with a few figures. Let us assume that the death rate in England and Wales was 30 in 1700, a rate roughly consistent with Scandinavian estimates for a few decades later. The population was 8.9 million in 1801 and 48.6 in 1971. Assuming that the birth rate was 40 between 1801 and 1831 and 35 between 1831 and 1841, and applying the national birth rates from 1841 to 1971, if the death rate had remained unchanged at 30 the population in 1971 would have been 7.1 million. The reduction of mortality was evidently responsible for the growth of population from the beginning of the eighteenth century, for if the rate had remained at its initial level, any increase in population due to a rising birth rate would have been almost eliminated by its later fall.

The estimate of population growth based on a constant level of mortality is, of course, theoretical. The death rate did in fact decline, and since the birth rate and death rate are not independent, it may be suggested that the initial reduction in mortality was secondary to a rising birth rate. However at a time when fertility was already high, an increase in births would have led to an increase in mortality if the latter were not falling for other reasons. This conclusion is based on investigations of the relation between infant mortality and maternal age and parity. I shall summarize the evidence.

In a general population of births, infant mortality rises with parity and is U-shaped in relation to maternal age; it is highest for the late children of young mothers. In England and Wales, in 1949, the rates were 37 and 24 for first-born of mothers aged 16–19 and 20–24 respectively and 84 for fifth-born of mothers aged 20–24.[7] During the eighteenth century, when mortality in infancy was much higher, the differences would have been far greater. In such circumstances mortality would inevitably have increased if the mean age of mothers at first pregnancy fell, say from 25 to 20, and mean number of children in families increased from five to six. In the effect on population growth the significant influence is not only the more frequent death of first-born children at the lower ages but the high mortality in the larger completed sibships.

The decline of the death rate between 1700 and 1838 was, therefore,

[7] Heady, J. A., Daly, C. and Morris, J. N. 'Social and biological factors in infant mortality. II Variation of mortality with mother's age and parity.' *The Lancet.* 1955, 1: 395–97

essentially a primary change. So, too, was its continued fall, for there was a large reduction of the age-specific mortality in most age groups. But even if this evidence were not available, we could hardly attribute a substantial and prolonged growth of population to the secondary effects of a falling birth rate.

Since a reduction in mortality was the predominant influence on population size in the past three centuries, the precise time when the increase began, and the relative contributions of birth and death rates in the initial phase (the first of the two issues referred to above), are not critical for our understanding of the growth of population as a whole. However, as pre-industrial changes have received so much attention, and their interpretation is frequently brought into discussion of the total period, it will be desirable to clarify one's viewpoint in relation to them.

The general conclusions drawn by a number of historians from work on pre-industrial societies are as follows. Animals in their natural habitats restrict fertility with regard for the resources of the environment so that mortality is kept at a relatively low level. Human societies also practise restraint, and Europeans in particular 'appeared to be reacting with a good deal of rationality along Malthusian lines of restraint long before the long-term decline in birth rates set in during the late nineteenth century.'[8] Studies of parish registers and of the demography of the aristocracy are believed to show that fertility was curtailed during most of the eighteenth century, and that it was the removal of restraint which led to the initial rise of population.

Although the exiguous data for pre-industrial societies provide some evidence of limitation of fertility, they are not sufficient to show the extent, duration or nature of the restrictions. I have already given grounds for believing that until the nineteenth century unconscious restraints on fertility from malnutrition and disease were more important than those that were consciously applied (contraception, abortion, prolonged lactation and the like); and that among conscious restraints on numbers, post-natal measures, particularly infanticide, were more effective than prenatal ones (see chapter 1).

These conclusions are consistent with the observation that both in the short term and the long term mortality is more sensitive than fertility to changes in economic and social conditions. It must also be remembered that during the seventeenth and eighteenth centuries, when fertility is thought to have been restricted, the birth and death rates were both about 30 and expectation of life at birth was nearer to 30 than 40 years. These rates are vastly different from those of developed countries today, which give us some idea of the levels at which numbers and resources can be said

8 Borrie, W. D. *The Growth and Control of World Populations*. London, 1970: 70.

to be in a reasonable balance. At the earlier levels Malthusian post-natal checks were clearly present, and it is incorrect to say that by limiting births 'pre-industrial west European populations managed to avoid the "positive" Malthusian solution of high mortality'.[9] Moreover, as Braudel has noted, when accounting for the demographic increase in China 'which was as marked and as undeniable as in Europe . . . one cannot point to any fall in the average age at marriage or leap in the birth rate.'[10]

I have concluded that the decline of mortality was the major influence on the growth of population during the past three centuries. However, the relative importance of changes in the birth rate and death rate is in a sense a technical issue, secondary to the question: What disturbed either rate? For, to the extent that fertility increased as a result of removal of restraints, it did so presumably in response to improvements in conditions of life; and believing that mortality was the predominant influence, I also conclude that it was amelioration of living conditions that led to its decline. The question remains as to the nature of the advances. If we believe that they operated chiefly through the birth rate, to account for the growth of population we are led to investigation of the relation between economic conditions and fertility; whereas if we conclude that the death rate was more important, our concern is with reasons for the decline of mortality. It should also be noted that if increased fertility were the major influence, we would need two explanations, one for the rise of population and another for the modern improvement in health. If reduced mortality were primary, the changes in population size and in health have a common cause, the reduction of deaths from infectious diseases.

The Transformation of Health

Although the documentary evidence is very unsatisfactory before births and deaths were registered nationally, there is no doubt that there has been a vast improvement in health during the last three centuries. During most of man's existence, it is probable that the majority of children died or were killed within a few years of birth. Such records as are available, taken with recent experience in developing countries, suggest that although there was considerable variation from time to time and from place to place, on the average, of 10 new born children, about 2–3 died before the first birthday, 5–6 by age 6 and 7 before maturity. In technologically advanced countries today, more than 95 per cent survive to adult life. For the first time in history a mother knows that the loss of one of her children before maturity

[9] Schofield, R. *Population Studies*. 1977, **31**: 180.

[10] Braudel, F. *The Structures of Everyday Life*. London, Fontana, 1985: 47.

is an unlikely event. The reduction of mortality is reflected in increased length of life: in 1700 life expectancy at birth was between 30 and 40 years; in 1982 it was nearly 75 for males and 80 for females in the country with the best figures (Iceland).

Figure 3.6 shows the death rate for males and females in England and Wales from 1841 to 1871. For the nineteenth century the rates are for the first six decades, and for the twentieth century they are for the first year of each decade; both are standardized in relation to the 1901 population to correct for the changing age structure, since with an ageing population the crude death rates underestimate the reduction of mortality which actually occurred. Throughout the period death rates were considerably higher for males than for females; they began to fall for both sexes in the eighth decade of the nineteenth century and the decline has continued to the present day.

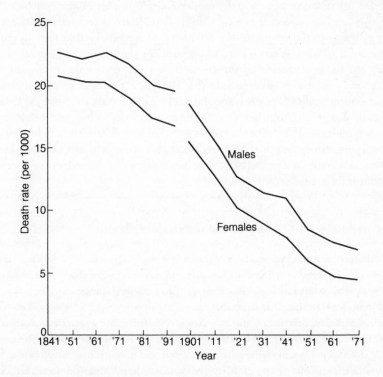

Figure 3.6 Death rates (standardized to 1901 population): England and Wales
Source: Role of Medicine: 31.

However, examination cannot be restricted to the nineteenth and twentieth centuries, since the decline of the death rate began well before

1838. Table 3.1 shows the proportion of the reduction which occurred in three periods: 1700 to the mid-nineteenth century (a third); the second half of the nineteenth century (a fifth); and the twentieth century (nearly half). These figures are based on the assumption that the death rate in England and Wales in 1700 was 30. The Swedish death rate for the period 1751 to 1800 was 27.4, and the rate for England and Wales is believed to have been at about the same level or a little higher.

Table 3.1 Reduction of mortality since 1700: England and Wales

Period	Percentage of total reduction in each period*	Percentage of reduction due to infections
1700 to 1848-54	33	?
1848-54 to 1901	20	92
1901 to 1971	47	73
1700 to 1971	100	

*The estimates are based on the assumption that the death-rate in 1700 was 30.
Source: McKeown, T. The Role of Medicine: 31. table 3.1.

When interpreting reasons for the decline of mortality we must rely to a considerable extent on national statistics of cause of death. Even today this is not a very reliable source of evidence. In an investigation based on a large series of patients who died in hospital in 1975 and 1976, clinicians' ante-mortem diagnoses were compared with the diagnoses made subsequently by post-mortem examination. The cause of death entered on the death certificate was seriously wrong in about a quarter of the cases.[11] The frequent errors in present-day certification, in spite of pathological, laboratory and other supportive evidence, raise doubts about nineteenth-century statistics, and still more about conclusions concerning diseases such as smallpox and plague in the eighteenth and earlier centuries when cause of death was not certified. The difficulties are particularly serious in pneumonia, where the evidence is prejudiced by changes in diagnostic fashions and in classification of cause of death. Scarlet fever was not separated from diphtheria in the national classification in England and Wales until 1855, nor typhus from typhoid until 1869. With due regard for such difficulties, something can be learned from examination of cause of death if the special features of individual diseases, and the considerable margin of error in the statistics, are taken into account.

Table 3.1 gives the proportion of the decline of mortality associated with infectious diseases, 92 per cent from 1848–54 to 1901 and 73 per cent from

[11] Waldron, H. A. and Vickerstaff, L. *Intimations of Quality. Ante-Mortem and Post-Mortem Diagnoses*. London, Nuffield Provincial Hospitals Trust, 1977.

1901 to 1971. On the assumption that there was no decrease in non-infective deaths before 1838 when cause of death was unknown, 86 per cent of the total reduction of the death rate from the beginning of the eighteenth century to the present day is attributable to the decline of the infections.

Reasons for the Decline of the Infections

We must now consider one of the most interesting questions in the history of human health. The predominance of infectious diseases as causes of death resulted from conditions created by the first Agricultural Revolution 10,000 years ago, when people began to aggregate in populations of considerable size. Why then did the infections decline from about the time of the modern agricultural and industrial revolutions, which led to the establishment of still larger and more densely packed populations? The answer to this paradox must be sought by examination of four possible influences: changes in the character of infectious diseases; medical treatment; reduced exposure to infection; and increased resistance to infection.

Changes in the character of infectious diseases   Was the decline of the infections during the past few centuries associated with changes in the character of the diseases? The relationship between micro-organisms and man is constantly changing as a result of the operation of natural selection on host and parasite, and there is no infection of which it can be said that there has been no change over a considerable period. Moreover, there is at least one disease, scarlet fever, in which this seems the best explanation for the variation in mortality observed in the nineteenth and twentieth centuries. Hence there is no difficulty in accepting that at any time some infections might be expected to increase in virulence, others to decrease, and still others to remain relatively constant.

Changes in the character of the diseases offer an explanation that has obvious attractions, and some historians have accepted it as main reason for the decline of the infections. Greenwood, for example, emphasized the importance of the 'ever-varying state of the immunological constitution of the herd',[12] and in his presidential address to the American Association of Immunologists, Magill wrote: 'It would seem to be a more logical conclusion that during recent years, quite regardless of our therapeutic efforts, a state of relative equilibrium has established itself between the microbes and the "ever-varying state of the immunological constitution of the herd" – a relative equilibrium which will continue, perhaps, just as long

[12] Greenwood, M. 'English death rates, past, present and future.' *Journal of the Royal Statistical Society*, 1936, **99**.

as it is not disturbed unduly by biological events.'[13] According to this interpretation, the trend of mortality from infectious diseases was due essentially to a change in the relation between hosts and parasites. The grounds on which it was possible to reach so radical a conclusion are interesting. Magill based his views on the ineffectiveness and dangers of vaccination against rabies, the decline of tuberculosis long before effective treatment was available, the behaviour of diphtheria in the nineteenth century (it increased in prevalence and malignancy in the middle of the century and declined before the introduction of antitoxin), and the rapid reduction of pneumonia death rates in New York State before the 'miracle' drugs were known, followed by an arrest of the decline from about the time when antibiotics were introduced.

But although this interpretation can be accepted for one or a few diseases, it cannot account for the fall in mortality from most infections during the last three centuries. To accept such an explanation we would have to believe that the modern transformation of health and growth of population were largely fortuitous, essentially independent of medical intervention and of the vast changes in economic and social conditions associated with industrialization. We would also need to explain why the advances in health were confined to the developed world.

Medical treatment   For many years the improvement in health and associated rise of population were assumed to be due to advances in medical treatment introduced progressively from the eighteenth century. This idea was proposed by Griffith, who was impressed by advances in medicine in the eighteenth century.[14] They included expansion of hospital, dispensary and midwifery services; notable changes in medical education; advances in understanding of physiology and anatomy; and introduction of a specific preventive measure, inoculation against smallpox. Taken together these developments seemed impressive, and it is scarcely surprising that Griffith and others concluded that they were mainly responsible for the improvement in health. This conclusion, however, results from failure to distinguish clearly between the activities of the doctor and the outcome for the patient, a common error in the interpretation of medical history. From the point of view of a student or practitioner of medicine, increased knowledge of anatomy, physiology and morbid anatomy are naturally regarded as important professional advances. But from the point of view of the patient, none of these changes has any practical significance until it contributes to preservation of health or recovery from illness. It is because there is often a considerable interval between acquisition of knowledge and

[13] Magill, T. P. 'The immunologist and evil spirits.' *Journal of Immunology*, 1955, **74**: 1.
[14] Griffith, G. T. *Population Problems of the Age of Malthus*. London, Frank Cass, 1967.

any demonstrable benefit to the patient, that we cannot accept changes in medical education and institutions as evidence of the immediate effectiveness of medical intervention.

What is needed is assessment of the contribution that immunization and therapy have made to the control of infectious diseases associated with the decline of mortality. This can be done only from the time when cause of death was certified. Since I have previously given a full account of such an enquiry,[15] I shall illustrate the approach and results by reference to the disease which contributed most to the reduction of deaths.

Respiratory tuberculosis accounted for 17.5 per cent of the fall of mortality in England and Wales between 1848–54 and 1971; more than half of this improvement occurred in the nineteenth century. Figure 3.7 shows the trend of mortality from the disease since 1838. The death rate fell continuously from 1838 when cause of death was first registered.

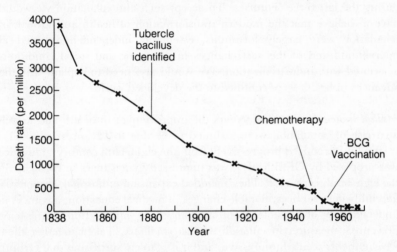

Figure 3.7 Respiratory tuberculosis: mean annual death rates (standardized to 1901 population): England and Wales
Source: as figure 3.1: 92.

The tubercle bacillus was identified by Koch in 1882, but none of the treatments available in the nineteenth or early twentieth century had a significant influence on the course of the disease. The many chemotherapeutic agents that were tried are now known to have been ineffective, as was also the collapse therapy practised from about 1920. Effective treatment began with the introduction of streptomycin in 1947, and immunization (by BCG vaccination) was used in England and Wales on a

[15] McKeown, T. *The Role of Medicine: Dream, Mirage or Nemesis.* Oxford, Basil Blackwell, 1979.

substantial scale from 1954. By these dates mortality from tuberculosis had fallen to a small fraction of its level in 1848; indeed most of the decline (57 per cent) had taken place before the beginning of the present century.

Figure 3.7 does, of course, obscure the large contribution treatment has made in the later stages of the epidemic. On the assumption that without streptomycin the decline of mortality would have continued at about the same rate as between 1921 and 1946, it was estimated that in the period since it was introduced (1948–71), chemotherapy reduced the number of deaths by about half by preventing deaths and restricting infectivity. But over the whole period since cause of death was first recorded (1848–71) its contribution to the reduction was 3.2 per cent.

BCG vaccination was used from about the same time as streptomycin, and it is therefore difficult to separate the effects of the two measures. In the examination of the trend of mortality it was assumed that the benefit was due wholly to chemotherapy. That this assumption is not unreasonable is suggested by the experience of the Netherlands, which has never had a national BCG programme, but nevertheless had the lowest death rates for respiratory tuberculosis of any European country in 1957–59 and 1967–69.

The history of tuberculosis illustrates, perhaps better than that of any other infection, a general point about the contribution of therapy to the reduction of mortality. Effective clinical intervention came later in the history of the disease, and over the whole period of its decline the effect was small in relation to that of other influences. But although the problems presented by tuberculosis in the mid-twentieth century were smaller than those in the early nineteenth, it was still a common and often fatal disease with a high level of associated morbidity. In two of its forms, tuberculosis meningitis and miliary tuberculosis, it was invariably fatal. The challenge to medical science and practice was to increase the rate of decline of mortality, and if possible, finally remove the threat of a disease which had been a leading cause of death for nearly two centuries. In this it was remarkably successful, and it would be as unreasonable to underestimate this achievement as to overlook the fact that it was preceded, and probably necessarily preceded, by modification of the conditions – low resistance from malnutrition and heavy exposure from overcrowding – which had made tuberculosis so formidable.

After reviewing the effects of immunization and treatment on the infections as a whole I summarize the conclusions as follows: 'Except in the case of vaccination against smallpox (associated with 1.6 per cent of the reduction of the death rate in England and Wales from 1848–54 to 1971), it is unlikely that personal medical care had a significant effect on mortality from infectious diseases before the twentieth century. Between 1900 and 1935 there was a contribution in some diseases: antitoxin in treatment of diphtheria; surgery in appendicitis; peritonitis and ear infections; salvarsan in syphilis; intravenous therapy in diarrhoeal diseases; passive immunization against tetanus; and improved obstetric care in prevention of puerperal fever. But even if these measures were responsible for the whole of the decline of mortality from these conditions after 1900, which clearly they were not, they would account for only a small part of the decreased deaths which occurred before 1935. From that time the first powerful chemotherapeutic agents, sulphonamides and, later, antibiotics, came into use. However, they were certainly not the only reason for the continued fall of mortality. I conclude that immunization and treatment contributed little to the reduction of deaths from infectious diseases before 1935, and over the period since cause of death was first registered they were much less important than other influences. In the light of these conclusions concerning the twentieth century, it is most unlikely that personal medical care had a significant effect on the trend of mortality in the eighteenth and early nineteenth centuries.'

Results which are broadly consistent with these conclusions have been obtained in the United States. McKinley and McKinley examined reasons for the decline of ten major infectious diseases and concluded: 'In general, medical measures (both chemotherapeutic and prophylactic) appear to have contributed little to the overall decline in mortality in the United States since about 1900 – having in many instances been introduced several decades after a marked decline had already set in and mostly having no detectable influence. More specifically, with reference to those five conditions (influenza, pneumonia, diphtheria, whooping cough, and polio-myelitis) for which the decline in mortality appears substantial after the point of intervention – and on the unlikely assumption that all of this decline is attributable to the intervention – it is estimated that at most 3.5 per cent of the total decline in mortality since 1900 could be ascribed to medical measures introduced for the diseases considered here.'[16]

Reduced exposure to infection I have noted (see chapter 2) that the predominance of the infections as causes of sickness and death was due in part to increased exposure in large human settlements. There were two main influences: crowding which resulted in more frequent contact, particularly with airborne infections; and unhygienic conditions which contributed particularly to the spread of water and food-borne diseases. To what extent was the decline of the infections in the industrial period attributable to removal of these influences?

[16] McKinley, J. B. and McKinley, S. M. 'The questionable contribution of medical measures to the decline of mortality in the United States in the twentieth century.' In: *Health and Society*, The Milbank Memorial Fund Quarterly, 1977, **55**: 405–28.

When considering this question we must distinguish clearly between the prevalence of a disease in the community and the mechanism of exposure to it. Tuberculosis, for example, was very common during the late eighteenth and early nineteenth centuries, and both working and living conditions under industrialization must have increased exposure to air-borne diseases. However, as the nineteenth century advanced its prevalence declined, while crowding continued and probably increased. It may, therefore, be said that there was no primary reduction of transmission of such disease as was present. But there was nevertheless a secondary reduction of exposure which resulted from the diminished prevalence.

The same trends must have occurred in the case of other air-borne infections. Exposure increased in the industrial towns, where populations expanded rapidly and working and living conditions were virtually uncontrolled. In the nineteenth century, house-building programmes did little more than keep pace with the increase in population size, and in England and Wales the number of persons per house fell only slightly, from 5.6 in 1801 to 5.3 in 1871. In the case of tuberculosis considerable importance has been attached to the segregation of patients in sanatoria. This may have been effective in the twentieth century, but it was probably insignificant in the nineteenth, for by 1900 only a few sanatoria had been provided by progressive local authorities or under voluntary auspices, and most patients were still admitted to Poor Law infirmaries.

In relation to the general interpretation of influences of the infections, the most significant conclusion is that in the case of air-borne diseases it was diminished prevalence which led to reduced frequency of transmission and not reduced ease of transmission which led to diminished prevalence. We must look elsewhere for the explanation of diminished prevalence.

It is in respect of water and food-borne diseases that the question concerning exposure is most important, for it is on the purification of water, efficient disposal of sewage and food hygiene that reduction of water- and food-borne diseases primarily depends. There are good grounds for thinking that at least the first two of these influences deteriorated in the first half of the nineteenth century. In a vivid essay, Chapman described the circumstances which led to a crisis in London's sewage disposal system in the 1840s.

The most apparent – and fundamental – precipitating factor was the increase in population. But Chadwick's zealous insistence on abolition of the cesspool was, paradoxically, an immediate precipitating factor. Prior to Chadwick's time, human excreta had been disposed of at or near the sites of their origin. Chadwick, by requiring the installation of flush toilets, moved the unwanted material well away from its myriad sites of origin, but gave insufficient thought to the effects of dumping such enormous quantities of sewage into the Thames in the London area. The result was the Great Stink, an infinitely more powerful stimulus to legislative action than Snow's work on transmission of cholera, or than the appallingly high death rates from the disease in the slum areas of east London, Southwark, Lambeth and Vauxhall.[17]

Although there may be doubts about the last point, there should be none about the main conclusion: the primitive sewage systems, which had served ineffectively in previous centuries, deteriorated rapidly under the pressures created by the greatly enlarged populations of the industrial towns. Their collapse carried its own risks and had unpleasant features; but, what was even more serious in relation to exposure to infectious disease, it led to further pollution of the sources on which the towns depended for their water. It was not until the second half of the nineteenth century that these risks were largely controlled, in London by new sewage systems and measures for purification of water supplies. But in the pre-registration period, and particularly its latter part, there is little doubt that exposure to water-borne diseases increased.

A substantial decline in mortality from intestinal infections began in the late nineteenth century, from the eighth decade in England and Wales and Sweden and somewhat later in most other developed countries. This advance coincided with improvements in public water supplies and sewage disposal, and it can confidently be attributed to the reduced exposure to infection which resulted from these changes.

We can be less certain about food hygiene in the same period. There was little if any improvement in milk, the most important component of the diet at that time as a vehicle for transmission of disease. It was not until the late nineteenth century that commercial pasteurization and bottling of milk was introduced, and not until the twentieth century that a safe supply became generally available.

Since most solid foods are protected from contamination, not by sterilization and sealing as in the case of milk, but by precautions in handling and distribution involving many people, it is not possible to say when the transition to a safer supply was achieved. Indeed outbreaks of food poisoning still occur in the most advanced countries. However, it seems unlikely that there was much improvement in food hygiene before the twentieth century; and indeed it may have deteriorated, since the growth of towns made it necessary to transport large quantities of food from rural to urban areas, with increased handling and delayed consumption.

This conclusion may be thought to overlook the contribution that personal hygiene has made to the advance in health. Standards were under-

17 Chapman, C. B. 'The year of the Great Stink.' *Pharos*, 1972: 90.

standably low in the eighteenth century, but are believed to have improved by the mid-nineteenth. Nevertheless they are unlikely to have contributed much to the decline of mortality, for it is the condition of water and food which mainly determines the risk of infection, rather than the cleanliness of the hands or utensils in which they are brought to the mouth. This point is well illustrated by the fact that in a developed country, where hygienic standards are good, a young child is relatively safe, although its hands, mouth and clothing are frequently contaminated, whereas in a developing country, where hygiene is poor, scrupulous personal cleanliness alone is ineffective, and an individual must seek protection from infection by boiling water or eating only cooked food. As a defence against diseases such as typhoid and cholera when the source is infected, the washing of hands is about as effective as the wringing of hands.

It is possible that there were minor improvements in the preparation and handling of food in the eighteenth and early nineteenth centuries. But national statistics indicate that the significant decline of infections caused by food began during the last years of the nineteenth century and coincided with substantial improvements in food hygiene, particularly in respect of milk. The high levels of infant mortality and of gastro-enteritis as a cause of death before 1900 in England and Wales, and their rapid reduction from that time, are impressive evidence of the period when food hygiene really advanced.

Increased resistance to infection   If the decline of mortality from infectious disease was not due to a change in their character, and owed little to reduced exposure to micro-organisms before the late nineteenth century or to medical treatment before the twentieth, the possibility that remains is that the response to infections was modified by increased resistance brought about by immunization or improved nutrition.

I have already referred briefly to the contribution of immunization to the control of smallpox, diphtheria and tetanus in the early years of this century; more recently effective protection has become available against several other infections, including measles, poliomyelitis, whooping cough and – more arguably – tuberculosis. But these measures came relatively late in the history of infectious diseases, and we must find another reason for the large reduction of mortality which occurred before 1935. The most credible explanation is that it was due to improvement in nutrition.

It should be said at once that there is no direct evidence that nutrition improved in the eighteenth and early nineteenth centuries. Evidence which would be regarded as convincing would be an increase in *per capita* food consumption or clinical evidence of improvement in nutritional state. These data do not exist, and few historical questions of such complexity would ever be resolved if they could be settled only by contemporary evidence of this kind. The case for the significance of nutrition is circumstantial, and in this it is like the case for the origin of species by natural selection.

The grounds for regarding better nutrition as the first and main reason for the reduction of infectious deaths are threefold: the explanation is consistent with present-day experience of the relationship between malnutrition and infection; it accounts for the fall of mortality and growth of population in many countries at about the same time; and when extended to include improved hygiene and limitation of numbers, it attributes the decline of the infections to modification of the conditions which led to their predominance.

The most useful evidence of the relation between nutrition and infectious diseases comes from the experience of physicians who have worked extensively with infants and children in developing countries. As already noted (see chapter 2) this experience leaves no doubt that although malnutrition has not the same effect in every disease, in general it is a major determinant of infection rates and of the outcome of infection.

The rapid growth of population in a large number of countries which differed in economic and other conditions has led some historians to conclude that no common explanation is likely to be adequate. The opposite conclusion seems more plausible: the widespread expansion of numbers in the same period of history in spite of variation in circumstances suggests the possible operation of a common major change. The increase in food supplies which resulted from advances in agriculture and transport during the eighteenth and nineteenth centuries was such a change. Its effect on population growth in a country would, of course, be determined by many variables, particularly the initial level of fertility and mortality, the subsequent behaviour of the birth rate and the amount of migration. Hence the variation in the timing and extent of the increase of numbers does not exclude the possibility that the reduction in mortality was first, and for some time, due to improvement in nutrition.

But perhaps the most important requirement in a credible explanation for the decline of infectious diseases is that it should have regard for the reasons for their predominance. We cannot be satisfied with an interpretation which suggests that the conditions which made the infections the common causes of sickness and death for 10,000 years remained essentially unchanged. This would be the case if immunization and therapy were the major influences during the past three centuries. It would also be true if mortality had fallen largely because of a reduction of virulence of micro-organisms. Moreover, if these were the reasons for the decline of the infections we could be anything but confident about the their future control. For in the light of experience of drug resistance we cannot predict the long-term consequences of immunization and therapy; and if deaths from infectious disease decreased because of a fortuitous change in virulence, they could quite readily increase again for the same reason.

The influences which led to the predominance of infectious diseases from the time of the first Agricultural Revolution were the expansion and aggregation of populations, poor hygiene and insufficient food; and I have attributed the decline of the infections to modification or removal of these influences spread over a century or more. During industrialization, however, the aggregation of populations increased; and in the early stages the hygiene, to put it cautiously, did not improve. It is, therefore, an impressive piece of circumstantial evidence, if no more, that a large increase in food supplies coincided with population growth in many countries which differed widely in economic and other conditions. (England and Ireland are remarkable examples.) Of course, it is arguable that the expanded population consumed all the additional food so that there was no increase in consumption per head. But in view of the other circumstantial evidence, as well as the lack of substance in alternative explanations, it seems more likely that at a time when the birth rate and death rate were high, the population expanded initially because better nutrition resulted in increased resistance to infectious diseases, particularly among infants and children.

Deaths from Non-infective Causes So far as can be judged from national statistics for England and Wales, nearly all of the reduction of mortality before the twentieth century resulted from a decrease of deaths from infectious diseases. However, there are two causes of non-infective deaths which are inadequately reflected in national statistics, infanticide and starvation. Infanticide was probably important until the last quarter of the nineteenth century. Various developments contributed to its decline – foundling hospitals, a rising standard of living and maternal and child welfare services; but the most important influence was probably the adoption of contraceptive practices, from the late nineteenth century, which prevented the birth of unwanted children. Although less common, food deficiency diseases and to be frank, starvation were other non-infective causes of death whose frequency decreased from the eighteenth century.

Non-infective conditions accounted for about a quarter of the reduction of the death rate in the twentieth century. Their decline was due to multiple influences. In several diseases therapeutic measures were effective: for example, surgery in treatment of accidents and digestive illnesses, and obstetric and paediatric services in the care of pregnant women and newborn children. But a substantial part of the advance resulted from other causes, particularly improvement of nutrition of mothers and children. Without attempting to rank them in order of importance, I conclude that the influences mainly responsible for the decline of mortality from non-infective conditions were contraception, medical treatment and improved nutrition.

Limitation of Numbers

In the preceding discussion, both the modern rise of population and the associated transformation of health were attributed essentially to the decline of mortality from infectious diseases. These were not the first major changes; the population of the world expanded after the transition to agriculture, and there were large increases in Western Europe between 1100 and 1350 and again between 1450 and 1650. However, these and many other less reliably recorded expansions of population and (presumably) improvements in health were all reversed in time. Only the modern changes have continued unabated: expectation of life is still increasing in developed countries, and most of their populations are rising, if at a somewhat slower rate.

The explanation of the difference from past experience is to be found chiefly in the behaviour of the birth rate. All previous advances were offset fairly rapidly by rising numbers, clear evidence that efforts to restrict population growth by control of fertility and deliberate killing were inadequate. Populations expanded to the size at which food resources were insufficient, and malnutrition led to increased mortality from infectious disease. Hence the improvements in health and expansions of population were in time arrested or reversed.

In the nineteenth century, however, apparently for the first time, there was effective limitation of births. It appeared first in France, where a marked decrease in the birth rate after 1789 is believed to have been due to the spread of contraceptive practices.[18] In England and Wales the decline was delayed until the eighth decade, but its significance in relation to health can hardly be exaggerated. If the birth rate had continued at its early nineteenth century level without a compensating rise of mortality, the population today would be about 140 rather than 50 million, with devastating consequences for health and welfare. Moreover the restraint on reproduction probably had a direct effect on mortality, since the virtual elimination of infanticide was due mainly to avoidance of unwanted pregnancies. The limitation of numbers was therefore the essential complement

[18] Braudel, F. 1985, *Structures of Everyday Life*: 55.

without which the advances in health would in time – and on an evolutionary scale, very short time – have been reversed.

The Price Paid for the Improvement in Health:
Non-Communicable Diseases

The changes in health which have arisen in association with industrialization are generally, and rightly, regarded as an improvement. In developed countries most people now have enough to eat; their drinking water is pure, or pure enough; sewage is dealt with cleanly and efficiently; the risks of exposure and death from air-borne infections are reduced by effective medical measures, and the risk of infection from food, although still present, is greatly reduced. For the first time it can be said that numbers and resources are in reasonable balance. But the decline of the infections has led to a new pattern of disease, most clearly reflected in changes in the common causes of death. Infectious diseases are no longer the leading causes, and cancer and cardiovascular disease in its multiple forms now account for about two-thirds of the deaths.

There are broadly two ways in which the new disease pattern might be regarded. It might be thought of as an underlying core of diseases, largely genetically determined, formerly obscured by the shortness of life and the predominance of the infections. This interpretation is consistent with the fact that the most important non-communicable diseases occur late in life and are uncommon in a young population. But the change in disease prevalence might also be due largely to the changes in conditions of life which have resulted from industrialization and the transfer from rural to urban life. Moreover, in relation to at least one of the most important influences on health (food), it is a short step from deficiency to excess.

In chapter 6, I shall discuss reasons for believing that the second is the more credible hypothesis, that the predominant causes of sickness and death in the developed world are due chiefly to conditions which have arisen in association with industrialization. Some are changes in the environment over which the individual has little control – atmospheric pollution, adverse working conditions and the like; others are changes in behaviour associated with, and in some cases encouraged by, affluence.

If the non-communicable diseases have arisen under the conditions which have led to the decline of the infections, they can be regarded as the price for the advance in health of the past two centuries. But is it a price that must be paid? Are the new diseases an inescapable consequence of the changes which led to the reduction of infectious deaths? To answer this question we must consider the origins of non-communicable diseases, and this subject will be discussed in chapter 6.

In summary: The transformation of health and rapid rise of population in the Western world during the last three centuries have a common explanation: they resulted from a decline of mortality from infectious diseases. The infections declined mainly for two reasons: increased resistance to the diseases due to improved nutrition; and reduced exposure to infection which followed the hygienic measures introduced progressively from the late nineteenth century. The contribution of medical treatment and immunization to the decline of mortality was delayed until the twentieth century, and was small in relation to that of the other influences.

The modern advance in health was not reversed by rising members, as it had been after the first Agricultural Revolution, because the nutritional and hygienic improvements were accompanied by a reduction of fertility. Population growth was restricted to a rate consistent with the requirements of health, and for the first time it could be said that numbers and resources were in balance, so that the Malthusian adjustment through high mortality was no longer applied.

However, a price has been paid for the improvement in health during the last few centuries: the infections have been displaced as the predominant causes of premature death by non-communicable diseases such as cancer and cardiovascular disease. Whether these diseases were a consequence of the changes which led to the advance in health, or were always present but concealed by the shortness of life and predominance of the infections, is a question to be decided in the light of knowledge of their origins.

PART II

Disease Origins

Introduction

I discussed Part I, the influences which have determined the extent and character of disease problems and the rate of population growth in the three major periods into which human experience can be divided. I concluded that in spite of the enormous diversity in the nature of diseases, the common causes of sickness and death were determined essentially by the prevailing conditions of life. I shall draw on the conclusions in Part II to examine the origins of disease, before considering (in Part III) the significance of disease origins for disease control.

In an operational approach to aetiology, where the aim is to find the best means of controlling disease, the most fundamental distinction that can be made between diseases is according to whether they are determined at the time of fertilization. For serious, untreatable conditions established at fertilization, unless the time comes when defective genes can be replaced, the only complete solutions would be selective avoidance of conception or elimination during pregnancy by abortion. In contrast, diseases which are not inevitable from fertilization could be prevented if it were possible to control the environmental (including behavioural) influences which are also required for their manifestation. This conclusion does not overlook the importance of the genes in such diseases: if the required environmental component is present, the frequency of a disease is determined by the genetic constitution of the population. Nevertheless, most people are affected only in the appropriate environment. This is as true of non-infectious as of infectious diseases, of lung cancer and cirrhosis of the liver as of tuberculosis and poliomyelitis.

Geneticists have understandably approached disease classification against the background of genetic interest. In a discussion of the 'new genetics' and clinical practice, Weatherall regarded as genetic disorders single gene defects, chromosomal aberrations, congenital malformations and other diseases to which genes contribute.[1]

There are some disadvantages in this classification. In the first place, it groups abnormalities (the single gene defects and chromosomal aberrations), for which the genes are both necessary and sufficient requirements, with others for which they are only a necessary requirement. The common malformations, and most of the 'other diseases' referred to (major mental disorders, coronary artery disease, rheumatoid arthritis and the like) are not inevitable from the time of fertilization, but are determined largely by other influences before or after birth. Secondly, since there is variation in susceptibility to all diseases, it can be argued that there is a genetic component in the aetiology of every disease. And thirdly, from an operational viewpoint the usefulness of the observation that there is a *strong* genetic component in the aetiology of a disease not determined at fertilization may be questioned, on the grounds that what matters in practice is not the strength of the genetic component but the feasibility of controlling the environmental influences. For example, the genetic component might be said to be strong in tuberculosis, to which some people are genetically much more susceptible than others; yet the disease declined mainly because of environmental measures – reduced exposure to infection and increased resistance due to better nutrition. The strength of the genetic component in the aetiology of diseases tells us little about the tractability and means of their control. In the discussion which follows I shall restrict the term genetic diseases to abnormalities determined at fertilization.

However, as a basis for discussion of disease control, it is not sufficient to divide the small number of abnormalities determined at fertilization from the much larger number that are determined later. One of the reasons for considering disease history (as in Part I) before disease origins, is that knowledge of the influences which have led to ill health in the past can suggest an operational classification. In the light of the conclusions reached in Part I, diseases will be divided into three classes, taking together all diseases manifested before birth (prenatal diseases), and dividing conditions manifested after birth according to whether they are due to deficiencies and hazards (diseases of poverty) or to maladaptation and hazards (diseases of affluence). By way of introduction, something should be said about each of these classes.

[1] Weatherall, D. J. *The New Genetics and Clinical Practice*, London, The Nuffield Provincial Hospitals Trust, 1982.

Prenatal diseases are considered separately from postnatal diseases because past experience suggests that they are essentially different in character; they have shown little response to the improvements in living conditions which have been so effective after birth. However, there are some disadvantages in this classification. In the first place, since our interest is in disease origins, we are concerned with the times and conditions under which diseases arise rather than the times when they are manifested. Yet an analysis of prenatal diseases is based on those that become evident before or at birth, and it therefore excludes some abnormalities determined before birth but manifested only in postnatal life, often in association with ageing. There is a second disadvantage, which results from taking together all prenatally manifested diseases: this brings into the same class genetic diseases determined at fertilization and others due to malnutrition, smoking and the like, influences which are similar to those that are predominant after birth. In later chapters I shall try to clarify these issues, but it is desirable at the outset to be aware that they exist, and that they arise from the decision that on balance it is best to consider all prenatally manifested diseases together.

In the present classification, postnatal diseases are attributed to 'deficiencies and hazards' (chapter 5) or to 'maladaptation and hazards' (chapter 6). (As noted above, they also include some genetic diseases determined at fertilization). The first term seems reasonably satisfactory for the common causes of sickness and death during most of man's existence, when hunter-gatherers lived in an environment to which, presumably, they were genetically well adapted, and early death was due mainly to shortage of basic requirements or hazards arising from search or competition for them. The same influences are still common today, particularly, but not only, in developing countries. Because they arise from lack of the essentials for life, it seems reasonable to regard diseases due to deficiencies and hazards as the diseases of poverty.

We are on less secure ground when attributing the conditions that have recently become predominant in developed countries largely to maladaptation. It is true that most of them have resulted from changes – in diet, exercise, smoking, reproduction and the like – which have led to maladaptation, changes to which human genes could conceivably adapt over a long period if natural selection were to operate unchecked by medical and other interventions. But the contemporary pattern of ill health in developed countries is also attributable to environmental hazards, some of which have resulted from industrialization (atmospheric pollution, pesticides), while others (warfare, homicide) have much in common with those of the pre-historic period (hunting accidents, tribal wars, infanticide).

Nevertheless, the recent profound change in disease pattern is a unique phenomenon in human experience, and it is clearly desirable to decide what the 'new' diseases are to be called. They have been referred to as diseases of civilization, diseases associated with industrialization, western diseases and diseases of affluence, and there is something to be said for and against the use of each of these terms.

The objection to attributing the diseases to civilization is that they have become common only in the last few centuries, in some cases in the last few decades, and the infections were still predominant in the high civilizations of Renaissance Italy, Elizabethan England and seventeenth-century France. Obviously our concept of civilization cannot meaningfully be based on health alone. Moreover, the impli-cation that countries in which the 'new' diseases are uncommon are uncivilized gives offence in the Third World.

The increased frequency of conditions due to maladaptation has coincided with industrialization, and they can be said to be associated with it. However, many of them are not directly attributable to industrialization, but are determined by its secondary effects (such as affluence). Furthermore, some are beginning to appear in developing countries which are not industrialized, as a result of western influences, including regrettably, sales pressure, as in the promotion of tobacco, sweet drinks and proprietary medicines.

The term western diseases has the advantage that it states where the diseases have occurred rather than why, but the disadvantage that some of the countries concerned are not western, and could equally well be described as northern; or temperate, if industrialized countries in the southern hemisphere are included. Moreover the non-communicable diseases are emerging in countries in Asia, Africa and Latin America, as the character of health problems changes under Western influence and with economic and industrial development.

For the purposes of the present discussion they will be called diseases of affluence, in contrast to those attributed to deficiencies and hazards which will be referred to as diseases of poverty. The terms are not entirely satisfactory: impoverished populations are increasingly exposed to risks of affluence (tobacco, alcohol, drugs and the like), and the people of developed countries are by no means all protected from the ill effects of poverty. However, the terms do specify the chief determinants of the character of health problems, the poverty which has been responsible for lack of the essentials for life, and the relative affluence which has created living conditions far removed from those for which human beings are genetically equipped.

Can all diseases be assigned unequivocally to one of the three classes? It is possible to think of some that would be difficult to classify, particularly in the field of mental illness. (For example, a suicide or manic depressive illness in a hunter-gatherer). However, the difficulty arises mainly from lack of knowledge of aetiology rather than from the deficiencies of the classification. There is no ambiguity in the statements that diseases are manifested before or after birth, and that environmental influences are divisible into those which expose a population to risks to which it is not genetically adapted and those, referred to as deficiencies and hazards, which prejudice the health of a population even in an environment to which it is well adapted.

4

Prenatal Diseases

Perhaps the starting point for examination of prenatal diseases should be recognition that they are much less tractable than those that are determined after birth. So far as we can judge, the frequency of the common and severe congenital disabilities – malformations and mental handicap – has not been significantly reduced during this century, and in developed countries the large reduction of mortality in infancy and childhood has had no parallel in a decline of prenatal deaths. Figure 4.1 shows the remarkable change in the distribution of deaths in England and Wales at different periods of life since the mid-nineteenth century. There has been a large reduction of postnatal deaths, particularly in early life, but little change in prenatal deaths, in spite of the decline of the stillbirth rate (whose contribution to the total of prenatal losses is not large). We must conclude that most prenatal deaths and congenital disabilities have not been controlled by the influences which have transformed health after birth.

At this point, however, we should consider an apparent contradiction in this conclusion about the problems of prenatal life. There is said to have been little change in their frequency in developed countries during the period when postnatal mortality has declined rapidly; yet it is evident that internationally there is considerable scope for prevention of low birth weight by improvements in maternal health and nutrition. Is it not probable that there were substantial prenatal advances in developed countries in the last few centuries when nutrition greatly improved?

The explanation of this contradiction is that improved maternal health which leads to increased birth weight has its impact partly on stillbirth rates (which have indeed declined), but mainly on sickness and deaths in infancy and childhood. It has little effect on the indices which are commonly used in assessing the trend of prenatal problems: prenatal mortality which is mainly from spontaneous abortions; and congenital malformations and mental defect.

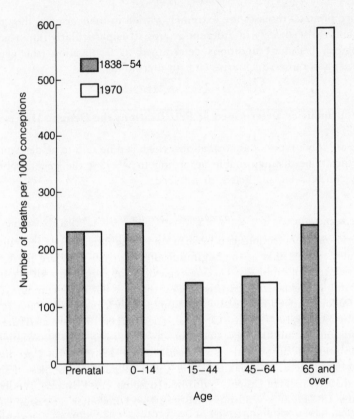

Figure 4.1 Mortality at different ages: England and Wales
Source: Role of Medicine: 22.

One other general point should be made before we turn to an examination of disease origins. When discussing prenatal and postnatal health problems together, we tend to think of deaths before birth (as we think of those after birth) as regrettable, and to assume that it should be the aim of medical research and practice to reduce their number. Of course among parents who badly want a child, particularly those who are infertile, there is understandable concern about the spontaneous termination of a pregnancy. But many pregnancies end almost as soon as they have begun, with no other evidence of their occurrence than a missed period; and in most spontaneous abortions which are early in pregnancy, the embryo or fetus is malformed. It must therefore be recognized that a considerable proportion of aborted embryos are abnormal at the time of fertilization or soon after, and their loss is both inevitable and desirable. Our chief concern is with infants who are born alive but seriously handicapped.

Since prenatal diseases are extremely varied in their origins, they must be examined separately in different groups. It is particularly important to distinguish between conditions determined at fertilization (the genetic diseases) and those which arise later in uterine life.

Abnormalities Determined at Fertilization: the Genetic Diseases

There are three types of abnormalities which can be said to be determined at fertilization, distinguishable according to whether the genetic abnormality can be seen, predicted, or inferred.

Chromosomal Aberrations

Chromosomal aberrations can be seen under the microscope, and current estimates suggest that at the beginning of pregnancy they are present in 7–10 per cent of embryos. Having regard to the complexity of events at fertilization, it is perhaps surprising that they are not more common. The large majority are eliminated by abortion, and their incidence in live births is about 5.6 per 1000 births. Of these, about 2 per 1000 are attributed to variation in the number of sex chromosomes, 1.7 per 1000 to variation in the number of autosomal chromosomes and 1.9 per 1000 to major chromosomal re-arrangements.[1] The well-recognized examples of these abnormalities include Down's syndrome (trisomy 21), Edwards' syndrome (trisomy 18), Patau's syndrome (trisomy 13), Klinefelter's syndrome (sex chromosomes XXY) and Turner's syndrome (the XO sex monosomic disorder).

In spite of intense interest in chromosomal aberrations for several decades, relatively little is known about their aetiology. The most striking observation was made long before chromosomes were discovered, an increase in the frequency of Down's syndrome at late maternal ages. The likelihood of recurrence in a sibship is also related to parental age, being greater for younger parents. A few other abnormalities show a less marked effect of parental age, but apart from these findings, the results from attempts to identify genetic or environmental influences causing chromosomal aberrations have been disappointing. Weatherall reviewed the evidence and concluded that 'it is difficult to see where we are going in research related to the aetiology of common chromosomal disorders'.[2] On the basis of present knowledge we start from the fact that they exist, with little information on why they exist.

[1] Weatherall, D. J. *The New Genetics*: 17.
[2] *Ibid.*: 19.

Single-gene Defects

These are the simply inherited abnormalities, dominant, recessive, or X-linked, whose distribution can be predicted on Mendelian principles. Where the fertility of those affected is low or absent, the frequency of the defective genes is reduced by natural selection, and the continued appearance of diseases such as haemophilia is attributed to new mutations. Phenylketonuria and a few similar conditions can now be treated with some success, and in time, no doubt, it will be possible to treat effectively some other single-gene disorders.

Estimates have been made of the frequency of single-gene defects, a task made more difficult by problems of diagnosis. In Northern Europe, autosomal dominants are said to occur in between 2 and 9 per 1000 births, autosomal recessives in about 2.5 per 1000, and X-linked disorders in a little more than 0.5 per 1000. However, there are large differences in the frequency of some conditions in different populations. Cystic fibrosis, for example, is found in 40–50 per 100,000 births in northern Europeans, and in only 1 per 100,000 in Afro-Americans and Orientals. Tay-Sachs disease is common in Ashkenazi Jews (17–40 per 100,000) but rare in Sephardi Jews and Gentiles (0.1–0.3 per 100,000). But much the most striking differences are in the frequency of thalassaemia (1000–2000 per 100,000 in Mediterraneans and Orientals, 5 per 100,000 in the United Kingdom) and sickle-cell anaemia (1000–2000 per 100,000 in Africans, 10 per 100,000 in the United Kingdom). Weatherall and Clegg concluded that the hereditary anaemias are probably the commonest single-gene diseases in the world population.[3] It is well known that thalassaemia and sickle-cell anaemia have achieved their high frequencies because the heterozygous carriers are protected against *P. falciparum* malaria, and it is possible that heterozygous advantage also accounts for the frequency of some of the other conditions in commonly affected populations.

In comparison with other types of abnormality, even with those which arise in the uterus, the single-gene defects are uncommon. Nevertheless they are responsible for a considerable volume of illness and large and increasing demands on health services. Hundreds of millions of people are carriers of the hereditary anaemias, and at least 200,000 severely affected homozygotes are born annually, approximately equally divided between sickle-cell anaemia and the thalassaemia syndromes. It has been estimated that about 100,000 infants with sickle-cell disease will be born in Africa each year, 1500 in the USA, 700 in the Caribbean and 140 in the UK.[4] The

[3] Weatherall, D. J. and Clegg, J. B. *The Thalassaemia Syndromes*. (3rd edn.) Oxford, Basil Blackwell, 1981.

[4] Weatherall, D. J. *The New Genetics*: 12, 13.

figures for thalassaemias are even more alarming, for the disease is widespread in Thailand, southern China, Laos, Cambodia, the Malay Peninsula and in localized areas of the Indian subcontinent. The thalassaemias also produce a major health problem in several Mediterranean countries. Even with inadequate therapy children live for two to four years, and with improved treatment the number surviving will increase. The burden on health services is large, and in Cyprus it was estimated that if all children with severe transfusion-dependent B thalassaemia were satisfactorily treated, in twenty years the health resources of the island would be consumed by the treatment of this disease.

Other Abnormalities Determined at Fertilization

Genetic disorders due to single-gene defects or chromosomal aberrations are observed in about 1 per cent of births. In most classifications other diseases, the large majority, are usually considered together as common diseases which are polygenic; most of them are not genetic diseases determined irreversibly at fertilization. The minority which are so determined are not associated with detectable abnormalities of single genes or chromosomes, and their inevitability from the time of fertilization can only be inferred. I refer particularly to certain diseases and disabilities of late life.

This interpretation rests on a conclusion which would hardly be disputed, that the maximum duration of life of a species is genetically determined. Of course it may be shortened by environmental accidents of many kinds; but it cannot be prolonged substantially beyond the normal span. Examples of exceptionally long lives of more than a hundred years are sometimes cited as evidence that life expectancy could be increased by internal or external measures; they prove only that like other characters such as stature and intelligence, the 'natural' duration of life is distributed over a wide range. The range could be modified by selective breeding if society were prepared to accept this objective and to introduce stringent control of reproduction in order to achieve it. Neither possibility seems desirable or likely.

If the maximum duration of life is determined at the time of fertilization, so too, it seems reasonable to believe, are some of the diseases and disabilities associated with its end. The programmed end is often preceded by a period of ill health, caused by the breakdown of non-essential organs, such as eyes, ears, or joints, or by the partial collapse of an essential one, such as the brain, the heart, or the kidney, usually from a vascular accident or deficiency.

However, it is easier to conclude that some disorders of late life are genetically determined than to specify the ones that are. It is not long since most of the ill-named degenerative diseases would have been labelled as inborn, or constitutional. It is now clear that cancer of the lung, chronic bronchitis, and some forms of heart disease are largely determined by environmental and behavioural influences, and it is probable that the same is true for many other diseases, including most cancers. Nevertheless it would be unreasonably optimistic to believe that all the disorders of the elderly are of this kind, and it is quite likely that some defects of brain, vision, hearing, and locomotion (for example) are the result of differential rates of wearing-out of organs determined at conception by genes.

The grouping of this third class of postnatal conditions whose genetic basis is obscure, with genetically determined prenatal diseases about which there is a good deal of knowledge, may seem unsatisfactory; and so it is, if we are concerned primarily with the underlying mechanisms. But if our interest is in disease control, the most useful distinction is between conditions which could be eliminated only by contraception or abortion, and those in which there is the possibility of prevention by environmental measures. It is on these grounds that some postnatal abnormalities, particularly in late life, deserve to be included among diseases determined at fertilization.

Abnormalities Determined after Fertilization

The majority of prenatal diseases and disabilities are neither simply inherited nor otherwise determined irreversibly at fertilization. They are usually described as multifactorial, by which is meant that they are caused by interaction between multiple genetic and environmental influences. All common diseases that have been studied are to some extent familial, and attempts have been made to attribute them to a few specific genes, or to a single gene of low penetrance whose effects are irregularly manifested. The results are unconvincing, and take us little beyond the conclusion that their genetic basis is obscure. The issues of most practical importance are the nature of the environmental influences which operate before birth and, in the light of their character, assessment of the feasibility of their control.

A number of prenatal abnormalities are due to well-recognized hazards such as iodine deficiency, smoking, radiation and infection, and clearly they provide scope for preventive measures. However, many of the common problems are not of this kind, and since they differ both in their origins and in possible means of control it will be desirable to consider them separately. I refer to congenital malformations, mental retardation and low birth weight.

Congenital Malformations

Estimates of the incidence of malformations in early embryos are unreliable, but Japanese observations on abortions leave little doubt that it is much higher than in live births. By combining observations on stillbirths and live births, the incidence of malformations in fetuses at the 28th week of gestation was estimated as 17.6 per 1,000 in a population of 94,474 total births. However, some malformations are not recognized at birth, and a follow-up to age 5 increased the estimate to 26.7. In this investigation a malformation was defined as 'an abnormality of structure attributable to faulty development'.[5] This working definition excludes conditions such as neoplasia and biochemical disorders when they are not accompanied by structural deformities.

Most congenital malformations are not determined irreversibly at fertilization. Malformations due to single genes are rare; those due to aberrations of chromosomes are common after conception, but many are eliminated by spontaneous abortion and, with the exception of Down's syndrome, they are infrequent among the malformed seen at birth. In the remainder, the majority, the genetical background is complex and obscure. It is known that many malformations, including the most serious ones, are established within a few weeks of conception, at about the time of implantation or during early embryonic development.

Even without precise genetical knowledge, there is a good deal of information about the likelihood of recurrence of malformations in a family in which a child has already been affected. After the birth of one malformed child the probability of another is increased, on the average, about ten times: to 1 in 50 for cardiac malformations and to 1 in 20 for malformations of the central nervous system.[6] A good deal of attention has also been given to influences such as maternal age, birth order, season of birth and social class. With the outstanding exception of Down's syndrome, where the increase with maternal age is striking, the relation to mother's age and order of birth is not marked, the common findings being a slight to moderate increase in frequency among first births and with increasing age, although some malformations show neither of these associations. Three abnormalities – congenital dislocation of the hip, anencephalus and patent ductus arteriosus – exhibit seasonal fluctuations, but the results are not consistent in all populations. Malformations as a whole appear to be

[5] McKeown, T. and Record, R. G. 'Malformations in a population observed for five years after birth.' *CIBA Symposium*, London, Churchill, 1960.

[6] McKeown, T. and Record, R. G. 'Congenital malformations of the central nervous system III. Risk of malformation in sibs of malformed individuals.' *Brit. J. Soc. Med.*, 1950, 4: 217–20.

unrelated to social and economic circumstances, although in this as in several other respects anencephalus is a notable exception, being more common in poor than in well-to-do families. Some remarkable geographical differences in frequency have been observed, particularly in malformations of the central nervous system, which are much more common in some countries (for example, Northern Ireland) than in others (France). The results from this approach have been interesting, in some cases striking; but with the exception of Down's syndrome they have not suggested any measures which would limit the frequency of conception of the malformed.

Particularly since the discovery of the fetal effects of thalidomide and rubella, many attempts have been made to identify teratogenic agents. There have been two main approaches. One is by investigation of teratogens in experimental animals: it has been possible to show that many physical, chemical and other agents can lead to malformations; but whether they do so in man – particularly in view of the high dosage or exposure in some experiments – is usually far from certain. The other approach is by assessment of influences that may have operated during pregnancies which were followed by the birth of a malformed child. Here the common difficulty is that mothers who have had an abnormal birth report a higher frequency of many occurrences than mothers whose children are normal. In a review of environmental teratogens, Smithells concluded that the evidence is acceptable in the case of thalidomide, steroid hormones, folate antagonists, alcohol, anticonvulsants, warfarin and some factor related to work in operating theatres.[7] For some of these the evidence leaves a good deal to be desired; and certainly if drugs such as alcohol and the anticonvulsants are teratogenic, they are clearly far less powerful agents than thalidomide. Rubella remains the outstanding example of an infective teratogen, although Dudgeon concluded that malformations may also be caused by cytomegalovirus, herpes simplex virus, varicella-zoster virus and Toxoplasma gondii.[8] However, except in the case of rubella, the malformations are uncommon in relation to the frequency of infections during pregnancy. Dudgeon found the evidence for an association with malformations unconvincing in influenza and respiratory virus, mumps and enterovirus. Whether mechanical influences in the uterus lead to congenital postural deformities is still an open question.

The problems presented by malformations from birth can be assessed by

[7] Smithells, R. W. 'Environmental teratogens in man.' British Medical Bulletin, London, 1976 32: 27-33.

[8] Dudgeon, J. A. 'Infective causes of human malformations.' British Medical Bulletin, London, 1976 32: 77-83.

considering their effect on the duration and quality of life.[9] It will also be convenient to examine the extent to which the results are influenced by medical treatment.

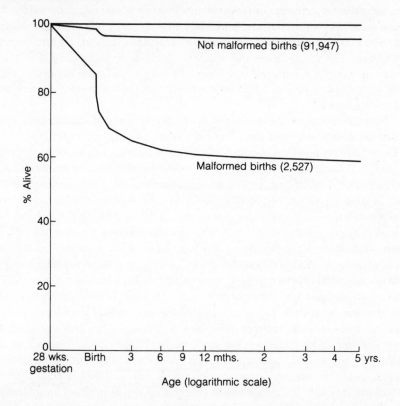

Figure 4.2 Survival to age 5 of malformed and not malformed births. Birmingham births, 1950-54

Source: McKeown, T. 'The Communities responsibilities to the malformed child'. *Proc. R. Soc. Med.*, 1967, **60**: 1219-24.

Figure 4.2 compares survival rates to age 5 of malformed and not malformed births. Mortality was very high immediately before and after birth, and the proportion surviving dropped to a little over 60 per cent by the middle of the first year. From this time, however, survival rates were not much lower than for normal births, and approximately three fifths were alive at 5 years.

[9] McKeown, T. 'The community's responsibilities to the malformed child.' *Proc. R. Soc. Med.*, 1967, **60**: 1219-24.

Assessment of the influence of malformations on the quality of life and of the effect of medical measures is more difficult, and can hardly be tackled without separate consideration of different abnormalities. I shall restrict attention to the common ones whose incidence in Birmingham in 1950–54 was above 1.0 per 1,000 total births (figure 4.3). Together they accounted for about two-thirds of all malformed births.

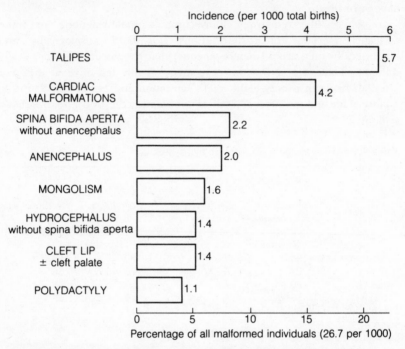

Figure 4.3 Incidence of common malformations. Birmingham births, 1950-54
Source: as figure 4.2.

Three of these malformations – talipes, cleft lip (with or without cleft palate) and polydactyly – can be dismissed in this context with little further comment. This is not to say that they are a trivial matter for those affected; or that if apparently unaccompanied by other more serious malformations they have no significance in relation to expectation of life. Indeed survival rates to age 5 are somewhat lower for children with cleft palate and lip than for not malformed births, possibly because of the presence of unrecognized internal malformations. But in comparison with the more serious conditions, talipes, cleft lip and polydactyly have relatively little effect on the duration or quality of life, and certainly they raise no question concerning the desirability of survival.

For quite different reasons this question also does not arise in anencephalus, one of the commonest abnormalities of the central nervous system. Over 90 per cent of those affected are stillborn, and the remainder die within a few days of delivery. Hence, unless some dexterous but misguided surgeon finds the means of prolonging the life of the anencephalic, the problems presented by this lethal condition will not extend beyond birth.

It is with the remaining four common malformations, or more accurately, groups of malformations (for both aetiologically and anatomically they are all heterogeneous) that assessment becomes really difficult. Table 4.1 shows the percentage of affected alive at different intervals between twenty-eight weeks' gestation and age 5. In relation to quality of life and the effect of medical intervention they must be considered separately.

Table 4.1 Survival to age 5. Birmingham births, 1950-54

	Percentage alive at age stated			
	Mongolism with or without cardiac malformation	Cardiac malformations without mongolism	Spinabifida with or without hydrocephalus	Hydrocephalus without spinabifida
28 weeks gestation	100	100	100	100
Birth	97	92	75	56
1 week	90	64	59	45
1 month	86	51	40	43
1 year	66	30	17	32
5 years	57	27	16	28
Number of cases	152	358	206	131

Source: McKeown, T. The communities responsibilities to the malformed child. Proc. R. Soc. Med. 1967, **60**: 1219-24.

Down's syndrome Early mortality is high, mainly because cardiac malformations are common, and only about two-thirds were alive at 1 year (table 4.1). From this age mortality was reduced, but it was still considerably higher than in normal births. Even so, probably at least half now survive to adult life, some to old age. Survival has so far been little affected by cardiac surgery, but it has undoubtedly been improved by the decline of infectious diseases which has resulted from better living conditions.

The life of the child with Down's syndrome is that of the mentally retarded, complicated in some cases by the presence of serious, usually cardiac, malformations.

Cardiac malformations In Birmingham in the period 1950–54 the proportions of individuals with cardiac malformations who survived to age 5 were 27 per cent for total births and approximately 29 per cent for live births (table 4.1). The latter is only about half the survival rate (60 per cent) given by Hay for Liverpool live births in 1960–64;[10] the difference is partly attributable to advances in treatment, but even more to a higher incidence of ventricular septal defect (for which mortality in the first 5 years is low) in Liverpool. To the extent that it reflects the substantial effects of improved treatment, the Liverpool estimate is probably a more accurate indication of the position.

Although there has been no detailed appraisal of the results of treatment, it is not difficult to assess broadly its probable overall effect on duration and quality of life. In a number of malformations – patent ductus arteriosus, coarctation öf the aorta, atrial and uncomplicated ventricular septal defects and pulmonary stenosis – operation offers the prospect of a normal life to patients who would die early if untreated. In Fallot's tetralogy the hazards of operation are greater, but results can be dramatic, leading to full activity. In other conditions, such as transposition of the arterial trunks, tricuspid atresia and aortic stenosis, where surgery is less successful, it is nevertheless worthwhile. Broadly it can be said that where surgery succeeds it usually restores the patient to what appears to be a normal life; unlike treatment of malformations of the central nervous system, it does not prolong the existence of patients who will remain permanently and seriously disabled.

Spina Bifida This condition raises, perhaps more acutely than any other, the difficult questions concerning the effectiveness and desirability of medical intervention.

Of 206 births with spina bifida, 75 per cent were live born but only 17 per cent were alive at one year; there was little further mortality before age five (table 4.1). The consequences of medical measures were investigated by Knox in 65,935 Birmingham births in the years 1960–62.[11] His conclusions were as follows.

There were 132 infants (liveborn and stillborn) with spina bifida; at four to five years after birth 13 were alive and well and 14 alive but disabled. With this incidence of disability, approximately two special school places were needed per 1,000 annual births. Knox examined the consequences of adopting either of the two treatment policies which might be favoured:

[10] Hay, J. D. 'Population and clinic studies of congenital heart disease in Liverpool.' *Brit. Med. J.* 1966, **ii**: 661.
[11] Knox, E. G. 'Spina bifida in Birmingham.' *Dev. Med. Child. Neurol. Suppl.*, 1967, **13**: 14.

1 Early operation upon children with no paralysis and no operations on other children. This would at least halve the number of disabled at five years, and would reduce the number of special school places to about 1 per 1,000 annual births.
2 Early operation upon all viable affected children. This would approximately treble the number of disabled and increase the special school places to about 7 per 1,000 annual births.

These estimates indicate that modern medical or surgical intervention offers a reasonably normal life to only a small proportion of these children who would otherwise have died or remained disabled. Moreover, the problem created for the medical and social, especially educational, services by the most active measures is potentially very considerable.

Hydrocephalus Hydrocephalus is probably more heterogeneous aetiologically than any of the other common malformations and many cases arise after birth from infection and trauma. So far as possible, postnatal cases were excluded from the Birmingham series (1950–54), and the 131 referred to in table 4.1 are the congenital hydrocephalics without spina bifida or encephalocele. Nearly half were stillborn and three quarters died before age five.

There has been no comprehensive assessment of the results of treatment, and the effect on duration and quality of life can be discussed only in general terms. Without surgical intervention approximately half of the liveborn hydrocephalics died within five years (table 4.1: effective treatment was not available in the period 1950–54). Most of those that survived suffered from some degree of brain damage, and Laurence and Coates reported that 37 of 82 surviving patients were severely handicapped.[12]

Appropriate surgical treatment increased the percentage of liveborn patients who survived, probably to over 75 per cent, and in early progressive hydrocephalus it often prevented or minimized further brain damage. Nevertheless, a considerable proportion of the patients saved by surgical intervention were seriously disabled, and they could not always be distinguished clearly at the time of operation from those who had little or occasionally, no disability.

Mental Handicap

In his classic discussion of the biology of mental defect, Penrose suggested that patients can be divided roughly into two classes, 'severe' and 'mild'.[13]

[12] Laurence, K. M. and Coates, S. 'Spontaneously arrested hydrocephalus.' *Dev. Med. Child. Neurol. Suppl.*, 1967, **13**: 4.

[13] Penrose, L. S. *The Biology of Mental Defect*. London, Sidgwick and Jackson, 1963.

This classification is consistent with Lewis' earlier division of the mentally handicapped into 'pathological' and 'subcultural' (or, as Penrose preferred, pathological and physiological) types.[14] As the names imply, the pathological cases are those in which diseases or pathological conditions are present; the physiological cases are apparently free from such abnormalities, and are mentally handicapped because they are at the lower end of the continuous distribution of intelligence in the general population. As would be expected, the two classes differ widely, not only in their aetiology, but also in their educational, social and medical needs.

Table 4.2 Causes of mental retardation in children

Severe mental retardation in children	
Known cause	%
Prefertilization: Genetic	
Chromosomal: Down's syndrome	32
other autosomal	2
sex-chromosomal* (average both sexes)	6
Monogenic	15
Intrauterine: environmental (maternal infection)	2
Perinatal: asphyxia/cerebral haemorrhage	7
Postnatal: meningitis/encephalitis/trauma/hypoglycaemia	2
	66
Unknown cause	
with congenital defect or dysmorphic features	14
with additional evidence of brain damage	10
without other abnormality	10
	34

*Recent data on the high incidence of the fragile-X syndrome may change this estimate.
Source: as table 4.1.

The mentally subnormal were formerly divided according to the level of intelligence as measured by I.Q.: feeble-minded (50–69); imbecile (20–49); and idiot (0–19). A large majority of the severe cases are pathological in the sense that disease is present. Lewis suggested that most of these cases were of environmental origin, but a different conclusion must be drawn from Carter's more recent analysis, based on three large surveys of severely handicapped children in hospital (table 4.2).[15] First, it should be noted that there was evidence of the presence of disease in 90 per cent of the cases.

[14] Lewis, E. O. 'Types of mental deficiency and their social significance.' *J. Ment. Sci.* 1933, *79*: 298.

[15] Carter, C. O. 'The aetiology of severe mental retardation in populations.' *Symposium on Recent Advances in the Field of Cytogenic and Biochemical Genetic Disorders Associated with Mental Handicap*, 1981, Bombay.

Fifty-five per cent were associated with genetic disease, either chromosomal or monogenic, and the high incidence of the fragile X syndrome may make the proportion even higher. The most common abnormality was Down's syndrome, which was present in about a third of these severely retarded children. Only 11 per cent were known to be due to environmental influences (infection, haemorrhage, asphyxia and the like) operating before, during or after birth.

However, most cases of mental subnormality, and, particularly mild cases, are of the 'physiological' type, in the sense that disease is not present. They are identified as handicapped, not according to an arbitrary and fixed level of I.Q., but by their inability to meet the educational, social and other standards set by the society in which they live. The more demanding these requirements are, the more common the abnormality will be, and in this sense the conditions in a society to some extent determine the frequency of mental subnormality. There is no biological or statistical justification for drawing a line between persons of normal intelligence and most of the mentally subnormal. The dividing line is a social one, determined by the extent to which the mental handicap interferes with the ability to lead a normal life.

Against this background it can be seen that the physiological types of mental subnormality are genetically determined in the same way as stature and body weight. That is to say they are largely due to genes which are multiple and additive; but they are also affected to a considerable degree by environmental influences. Children may become educationally retarded as a result of lack of parental interest or ability, emotional disturbance, irregular school attendance and frequent changes of school, as well as because of limited intellectual ability which is genetically determined.

In view of the large differences between severe and mild types of mental handicap, it is desirable to consider separately the medical and social problems which arise in relation to their care. In England and Wales severe cases were uncommon (.25 per cent in the general population) and many of them (25 per cent) were in hospital; mild cases were relatively common (2 per cent) and few (about 3 per cent) were in hospital.[16] Most severe cases have associated disease – often malformations; mild cases may have behavioural disorders, but their mental defect is primary rather than a secondary consequence of physical abnormality. It follows that the severe pathological cases would in principle have normal intelligence if their physical disease could be prevented or successfully treated; in the mild physiological cases the problems arise mainly from behavioural disorders or in relation to education, training and care.

[16] Penrose, L. S. *Biology of Mental Defect.*

Low Birth Weight

At the outset it is important to distinguish the problems of low birth weight in abnormal infants from those that arise in normal births. When a fetus is affected by an abnormality such as anencephalus or Down's syndrome, birth weight is low, in the former mainly because of early onset of labour, in the latter because fetal growth is retarded. But the formidable ethical and other issues related to the care of the malformed result from their abnormalities rather than their weights, and as they will have been discussed in relation to malformations they will not be considered here.

Most not malformed infants with low birth weights can be divided broadly into two classes, according to whether the reduction is determined essentially by internal causes such as multiple pregnancy, birth rank and early onset of labour, or by external influences of which the most important is insufficient food. In developed countries, where maternal nutrition is usually good, the sources of low birth weight are mainly internal; nevertheless, there are minority groups living in or near to poverty, in which low birth weight is due to maternal ill health caused largely by poor nutrition. In the Third World, the common substantial reductions in weight are almost always due to this cause.

Internal influences Since they throw a good deal of light on sources of variation in birth weight, it will be convenient to consider first the internal influences. It has long been considered necessary to identify small births which need special attention, and from about 1920 infants weighing less than 2500g were considered to be premature. This practice was open to criticism on two counts: as an administrative device for recognizing vulnerable infants, the limit of 2500g was too high; and since low birth weight may result from either or both retarded fetal growth and early onset of labour, identification of maturity with weight confused two different classes of problems. Subsequently, by international agreement, the definition of prematurity was changed. But in the meantime another term had appeared in the literature; 'intrauterine growth retardation' began to be referred to as an entity, in much the same way as 'premature birth' in the earlier period. The new term clearly distinguished low birth weight due to retarded fetal growth from that associated with short gestation, but it had the disadvantage that it tended to confuse the large number of different influences – fetal abnormalities, physiological causes, maternal malnutrition – which may affect the growth of the fetus.

A good deal has been learned about the various influences on birth weight from the study of multiple pregnancy, in which low birth weight is due partly to early onset of labour, but mainly to retarded fetal growth (fig. 4.4).[17] It is evident that in multiple pregnancy:

a Mean fetal weight is independent of the number of fetuses until about the 27th week of gestation.

b The rate of growth of multiple fetuses is slower than that of single fetuses from a stage of gestation which varies with the number: quadruplets from 26 weeks; triplets from 27 weeks; twins from 30 weeks. In the case of singletons, fetal growth is linear between 30 and 36 weeks; after 36 weeks the rate of growth is reduced.

c At the times when the rates of fetal growth are retarded, mean litter weights of twins, triplets and quadruplets are approximately the same – about 7 lb. The mean weight of single births at 36 weeks (when growth begins to be retarded) is 6.5 lb.

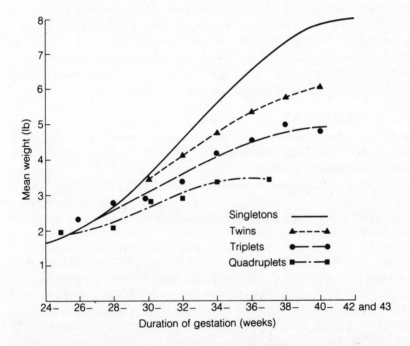

Figure 4.4 Mean birth weight of single and multiple foetuses related to duration of gestation. (Cubic curves fitted by the method of least squares)
Source: McKeown, T. and Record, R. G. 'Observations on foetal growth in multiple pregnancy in man.' *J. Endocrin*, 1952, **8**: 386-401.

[17] McKeown, T. and Record, R. G. 'Observations on fetal growth in multiple pregnancy in Man.' *J. Endocrin.* 1952, **8**: 386–401.

These results suggest that fetal growth can be supported in multiple pregnancy without prejudice to the individual fetus until the aggregate fetal weight reaches about 7 lb. It can also be shown that above this weight, litter weight increment is approximately the same for every size of litter.

There is no reason to suppose that the variation in growth rates of multiple fetuses is determined by fetal genes, and it must be attributed to maternal causes. What is less evident is the reason for the retardation which also occurs in the growth of single fetuses from 36 weeks (fig. 4.4). It might be determined by the fetal genes, or by the limitations that are imposed by the uterus in multiple pregnancy.

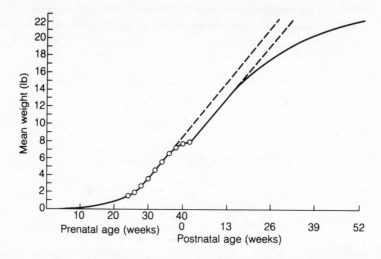

Figure 4.5 The prenatal (o) and postnatal growth rates of human singletons
Source: McKeown, T. 'Prenatal and early postnatal influences on measured intelligence'. *Brit. Med. J.*, 1970, **3**: 63-7.

That the latter is the explanation is evident from a comparison of prenatal and postnatal growth rates of single births (fig. 4.5).[18] After adaptation to the postnatal environment, the single infant resumes approximately the rate of growth shown by the fetus during the period of maximum growth between 30 and 36 weeks gestation. The genetically determined retardation does not occur until between three and six months after birth.

From both experimental and clinical observations it is known that the ability of the uterus to support the growth of the fetus is determined largely by maternal size. In human pregnancy, mean birth weight is related to the

[18] McKeown, T., Marshall, T. and Record, R. G. 'Influences on fetal growth.' *J. Reprod. Fert.*, 1976, **47**: 167–81.

size of the mother but not to the size of the father. From this and other evidence, it is clear that normal fetuses vary considerably in their rates of prenatal growth, according to their genes (related to the size of both parents) and to the resources of the uterus (related to the size of the mother). Two examples are shown diagramatically in fig. 4.6.[19] The growth of first born males with small mothers and large fathers (a combination of influences which maximizes fetal capacity for growth and minimizes maternal ability to support it) is compared with that of later-

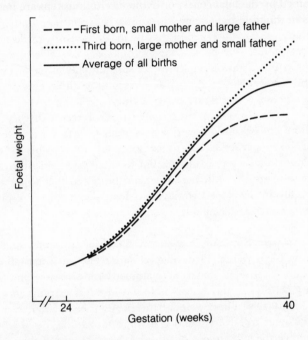

Figure 4.6 Two contrasting examples of human foetal growth
Source: McKeown, T., Marshall, T. and Record, R. G. 'Influences on foetal growth'. J. Reprod. Fert., 1967, **47**: 167-81.

born females with large mothers and small fathers (a combination which reverses the major influences). Fetal growth is likely to be considerably restricted in the first example and relatively unrestricted in the second. In respect of the probability of retarded growth, most normal single fetuses fall between these extremes, and are represented by the sigmoid growth curve shown as a solid line in fig. 4.6. The curve is, of course, a mean based on many different patterns, and does not necessarily correspond to the growth of any one fetus.

[19] McKeown, T., Marshall, T. and Record. R. G. Influence of pre-natal environment.

Does the child experience any ill effects in postnatal life in consequence of the retarded fetal growth which commonly occurs in both single and multiple pregnancy in developed countries? There are two lines of evidence which suggest that it does not. One is the observation that if postnatal conditions are favourable, the weight deficiencies are rapidly eliminated after birth.[20] The other is the finding that the retardation in single pregnancy, and the more pronounced retardation in twin pregnancy, have little influence on measured intelligence. This conclusion is based on the very small differences in verbal reasoning scores at age eleven, between sibs of different birth weights and durations of gestation; and, still more convincingly, on the observation that twins whose co-twins do not survive beyond one month after birth score almost as well as single births, whereas when both twins survive their scores are substantially lower.[21] This finding can hardly be explained except as a result of differences in postnatal experience between single and paired twins.

A more serious problem is presented by children with very low birth weights born after gestations of 27 weeks or less. Formerly few were treated and most were regarded as abortions; but today it is possible to keep many such children alive. The issues related to their care and survival will be discussed in chapter 7, but here it should be noted that so far they have arisen mainly in developed countries, where the requisite resources and clinical experience are available.

External influences   Smoking is probably the chief environmental determinant of low birth weight in developed countries, but internationally the most frequent cause is maternal malnutrition, common and severe in developing countries, and still to be found in a less extreme form in most developed countries. These weight deficiencies arise in children of mothers living in or near to poverty, and it is important to decide to what extent they prejudice the subsequent health and development of the children.

The answer depends to some extent on the degree of reduction of weight. In Birmingham a few years ago it was found that in children of immigrant mothers the mean birth weight was lower on the average by a few hundred grams. From the experience of normal births outlined above, it is unlikely that differences of this order would be significant in later life if the postnatal environment were satisfactory. The importance of this reduction of birth weight is not that of itself it seriously prejudices health and development,

[20] Cawley, R. H., McKeown, T. and Record, R. G. 'Influence of the pre-natal environment on post-natal growth.' *Brit. J. Prev. Soc. Med.* 1954, **8**: 66–9.

[21] Record, R. G., McKeown, T. and Edwards, J. H. 'An investigation of the differences in measured intelligence between twins and single births.' *Ann. Hum. Gen. Lond.*, 1970, **34**: 11–20.

but that it occurs in families in which postnatal conditions are likely to be unfavourable.

The extreme reductions of weight which occur in the Third World are another matter. Nevertheless, recent experience with very low weight babies in technologically advanced countries suggests that if medical care is adequate, and if postnatal conditions are good, most of these children develop normally and apparently without significant disabilities. In developing countries, unfortunately, neither of these requirements is met.

Conclusions

The separation of prenatal from postnatal diseases may seem to imply that the causes of disease before and after birth are always different. Clearly, they are not. Some prenatal abnormalities are due to influences such as food deficiency, alcohol and tobacco which are also important after birth; and some diseases and disabilities manifested after birth, particularly in late life, are determined at or soon after fertilization. The reason for separating prenatal and postnatal diseases is that the latter was due mainly to deficiencies and hazards or maladaptation, whereas most of the former are determined at conception or early in uterine life. The two classes are therefore essentially rather than invariably different, both in their origins and in their potential means of control. We know a good deal about the prevention of postnatal diseases but relatively little about the solution of most prenatal problems.

Prenatal diseases can be divided broadly into three classes, according to whether the abnormalities are determined at fertilization, during implantation and early embryonic development, or later in uterine life.

The conditions determined at fertilization are mainly the single-gene defects and chromosomal aberrations. They are usually manifested by the time of birth, but they include some postnatal conditions, particularly associated with ageing, which are also independent of environmental and behavioural influences. These abnormalities are correctly described as genetic diseases, since their defective genes and chromosomes are a sufficient as well as a necessary requirement for their existence. If estimates which suggest that between 7 and 10 per cent of embryos have abnormal chromosomes are correct, most genetic diseases are eliminated (fortunately) by spontaneous abortion. Nevertheless they are responsible for some congenital malformations, for most cases of severe mental subnormality, and for single-gene defects such as cystic fibrosis, Tay-Sachs disease and the hereditary anaemias, which reach high frequencies in certain populations.

The second class of prenatal diseases consists of those that are not established irreversibly at fertilization, but arise early in uterine life, probably from hazards associated with implantation and embryonic development. They probably include most malformations and some types of mental subnormality. In such cases the precise nature of the hazards is usually unknown and they may prove very difficult to identify and control.

The other abnormalities which arise during uterine life are quite different, in that they result from well recognized and largely preventable causes. Among malformations they include those due to rubella and thalidomide; and the variation in the variation in the incidence of anencephalus (by country of birth, season, social class and birth order) strongly suggests that it may be preventable, although the adverse influences have not yet been identified. Some diseases of children are due to iodine deficiency during pregnancy – cretinism, deaf mutism, spastic gait and feeble mindedness; others are caused by radiation and, possibly, alcohol, tobacco and drugs. But probably the most important, certainly the most common of the preventable conditions determined before birth, is 'low birth weight'. As currently used this term does not refer to an entity, since it includes at least three different types of problems: very early births, some of which are abnormal and would formerly have been regarded as abortions; births with small or modern weight reductions from physiological causes such as multiple pregnancy; and births of low weight due to maternal causes such as ill-health, malnutrition and smoking.

Although the origins of prenatal diseases are extremely varied, it is possible to draw some general conclusions about the nature of the problems they present. Perhaps the most important is that diseases in the first two classes are unlikely to be prevented by environmental measures, in the first, because they are established at fertilization, and in the second because the adverse influences occur very early in pregnancy when they are relatively inaccessible. This is not to say that they offer no scope for prevention and treatment. The prevention of rhesus haemolytic disease is a remarkable example of an advance made possible by a combination of genetic and clinical knowledge. The recognition and abortion of a fetus affected by Down's syndrome is another approach to an apparently intractable problem. Equally impressive in a quite different way is the immense technical accomplishment which restores a child with patent ductus arteriosus or atrial septal defect to a life of normal duration and quality. But for medical research the significant conclusion is that most diseases in these classes are unlikely to be prevented by control of environmental and behavioural influences, and they must be tackled by other means which depend on knowledge of their mechanisms. This indeed is the field which uniquely requires the traditional laboratory and clinical approaches, and the more successful other measures are in dealing with preventable conditions, the more important the residual problems established at conception or early in pregnancy will be seen to be.

The diseases due to well recognized hazards - iodine deficiency, smoking, radiation, infection and the like - clearly provide scope for preventive measures. The large problem of low birth weight is, probably necessarily, approached from two different directions. In specialized centres in developed countries improved clinical care is leading to the survival of a considerable number of low birth weight infants. Even more important, however, are attempts to improve maternal health before and during pregnancy, in order to reduce the frequency of low birth weight. In the same context we should also recognize that in several countries maternal mortality is still far above an acceptable level. Indeed in countries where maternal mortality is very high its true level is usually unknown, because there is no record of the number of pregnancies or of the number of deaths.

5

Diseases of Poverty

Diseases due to Deficiencies and Hazards

I suggested in Part I that a pivotal question in the history of human health is whether, by restraints on numbers population size was in general maintained at a level that the resources of the environment, particularly the food supply, could support. Since infanticide was probably the most effective means of limiting population growth the question might almost be rephrased by asking whether in the inglorious past parents were prepared to kill their children in order to maintain a tolerable existence, or only when driven by extreme necessity to reduce their numbers. After reviewing the evidence I concluded that population growth was not effectively restricted, and that until the nineteenth century man was no exception to Malthus' generalization that 'the tendency of all animated life is to increase beyond the nourishment prepared for it'. The consumption of unfamiliar foods, the search for new territories and finally, the transition to a more productive form of life under agriculture, were all motivated by the need for food.

This conclusion has a large bearing on interpretation of the determinants of health and disease. Our predecessors lived in an environment to which they were well adapted through natural selection, and they were largely free from disease due to maladaptation or defective genes. Even food deficiency was probably met to some extent by genetic selection of people who could survive on low food intakes, the ancestors of the unfortunates who today have to reduce their daily consumption to a few hundred calories in order to lose weight. But beyond a certain point lack of food could not be countered by genetic adaptation, and ill health was due mainly to the direct and indirect effects of food deficiency. As direct effects I refer to starvation and malnutrition; as indirect effects to hazards due to the conditions of life and, to the extent that it is influenced by nutrition and infectious disease.

Until 10,000 years ago the hazards from conditions of life were considerable. For hunters and gatherers trauma was a common cause of injury and death, the nature of the injuries being determined largely by the character of the habitat: Eskimos were at risk from cold and drowning, the Aborigines from fractures, the Siriono from falls from trees. Of course not all hazards were food related, and some human beings have always been ready to injure to kill their fellows or themselves for love or hate or for no apparent reason. But with due regard for such exceptions, the environmental risks to which hunter-gatherers were exposed were determined mainly by the nature of the habitat, which depended on the source and availability of food.

As previously noted (see pp. 29–40), conditions in the Pleistocene epoch were unsuited to the spread of human infectious diseases. Hunter-gatherers lived an open air, nomadic life in small groups, meeting only a few hundred people in a lifetime. Under such conditions most of the diseases which were later predominant could not have existed, and infection was due mainly to the zoonoses (which have other animal hosts), to commensals (such as the helminths) and possibly to a few human infections (such as tuberculosis and chicken pox) characterized by latency and recurrent disease. Response to such infections must have been determined substantially by the general state of health which in turn was influenced by nutrition.

The food provided by agriculture made it possible for numbers to expand; but as fertility was not effectively controlled, they expanded to the size at which food resources again became marginal. It is hardly possible to read an account of everyday life in the past without being acutely aware of the frequency and devastating effects of famine. As recently as the period between the fifteenth and eighteenth centuries the world consisted of one vast peasantry, and 'the rhythm, quality and deficiency of harvests ordered all material life'.[1] 'Famine recurred so insistently for centuries on end that it became incorporated into man's biological regime and built into his daily life. Dearth and penury were continual, and familiar even in Europe, despite its privileged position.' 'Things were far worse in Asia, China and India. Famine there seemed like the end of the world.'[2] It is on such grounds that it seems justified to conclude that the direct effects of food deficiency – starvation and malnutrition – were major determinants of disease and death in the historical period, at least until the nineteenth century.

But the indirect effects of food shortage were also important. After the introduction of agriculture and a more settled way of life, some physical hazards were probably reduced; but those due to infectious diseases were greatly increased, particularly after the establishment of cities about 5000 years ago. With large populations, living in unhygienic conditions, the

[1] Braudel, F. *The Structures of Everyday Life*. London, Fontana Press, 1985: 49, 73, 76.
[2] *Ibid.*

human infections which have no other animal host became the predominant causes of sickness and death. In chapter 2 I discussed reasons for
thinking that although the effects of malnutrition are not the same in every
disease, it has a profound influence on the frequency and seriousness of
infection. Perhaps the most persuasive evidence for this conclusion is the
fact that mortality from infectious diseases declined rapidly in some
countries in Europe in the nineteenth century when nutrition improved,
although there was little vaccination, no effective treatment, and exposure
to infections in the industrial towns initially increased.

Conclusions concerning the origins of human diseases before the
eighteenth century turn largely on the answers to two questions: Were
numbers in general maintained at a level that food resources could support?
And was experience of infectious diseases determined mainly by conditions
of life, particularly by the food supply, or was it essentially fortuitous, that
is independent of identifiable environmental or medical influences? We can
see that the answers to these questions are closely related. If food was
adequate, the high mortality and slow rate of population growth must be
attributed largely to the fortuitous behaviour of the infections; but if food
was seriously deficient, they can be explained credibly by its direct and
indirect effects. I concluded that for almost the whole of human existence,
disease and early death resulted mainly from basic deficiencies, or from
hazards related to them.

After the introduction of agriculture, the causes of sickness and death
resembled those of the hunter-gatherer period in that food deficiency was
still critical, but differed in that its effects were manifested largely through
response to infectious disease. In these circumstances an increase in food
supplies became a necessary requirement for a substantial reduction of
mortality, and limitation of numbers would have to coincide or follow if the
reduction was to be maintained.

As we have seen, these, with hygienic measures, were the critical
advances made in the last three centuries. The increase in food resulted
from advances in agriculture that spread through the Western world from
about the end of the seventeenth century. Improvements in hygiene were
initiated in the second half of the nineteenth century by sanitary reformers,
and greatly extended by the understanding of the nature of infection
provided by medical science. Limitation of numbers followed the decline of
the birth rate, which fortunately began in the same period (indeed in the
same decade in England and Wales), as the hygienic measures. It is one of
the remarkable coincidences of history that the indispensable control of
numbers appeared at precisely the time needed to ensure that the most
important advances ever made in human health were not lost.

As a result of these advances, diseases due to deficiencies and related hazards are no longer the principal causes of sickness and death in technologically advanced countries. In much of the world, however, the picture remains essentially unchanged. In this chapter I shall examine reasons for believing that they are still the predominant influences on health in the Third World, and that they remain important in industrial countries. I shall also consider the relation between poverty and health.

The Third World

'Do not waste your time on Social Questions. What is the matter with the poor is Poverty.' Bernard Shaw's pronouncement on conditions in the early twentieth century applies even more forcefully in developing countries today. To anyone who has travelled extensively in their rural areas where most people live, it will seem unnecessary to give much attention to the question of whether ill health is due to deficiencies and hazards rooted in poverty. Many children are visibly malnourished; sanitary conditions are primitive; drinking water is unclean; the food displayed in open markets is contaminated; and the number of people competing for the means of life is clearly excessive. Indeed, an analysis of disease origins, based on appraisal of the major influences on health in the past, may seem a circuitous route by which to arrive at the self evident conclusion that the most elementary requirements for health are that people must have enough to eat and they must not be poisoned. (A good deal of our knowledge of the determinants of health is epitomized in this simple statement.) It is therefore, perhaps, less necessary to demonstrate the importance of deficiencies and hazards than to assess their frequency and causes in the present day. They have been examined in numerous reports by international agencies such as the World Bank, The United Nations and the World Health Organization, and I shall summarize conclusions that have been drawn in relation to the critical influences: food, drinking water, sanitation and control of numbers.

Food

A World Bank study of the relation between poverty and hunger quoted an edict by the Emperor Wen in 113 BC: 'Why is the food of the people so scarce? . . . Where does the blame lie?'[3] The deficiency is even more remarkable today, because in many countries and in the world as a whole food supplies are believed to be adequate. The World Bank study concluded: 'The often predicted Malthusian nightmare of population outstripping food

[3] World Bank Policy Study. *Poverty and Hunger*. Washington, D. C. 1986.

production has never materialized. Instead, the world faces a narrower problem: many people do not have enough to eat, despite there being food enough for all. This is not a failure of food production, still less of agricultural technology. It is a failure to provide all people with the opportunity to secure enough food – something that is very hard to do in low-income countries'. Although one would question the statement that population growth has *never* outstripped food production, it is an accurate assessment of the position in many countries today.

In relation to health our interest is in the frequency of malnutrition and the reasons for its occurrence when food supplies are adequate.

In the last thirty-five years food production has increased dramatically, largely as a result of technological advances: the use of chemical fertilizers has increased 10 times; the use of pesticides 33 times; the amount of irrigated land has doubled; and high yielding disease resistant seeds have been introduced. Because of geographical, climatic and other differences, the technology has varied in different parts of the world. In Africa and Latin America there have been substantial additions to the arable area; in Latin America two-thirds of the increase in output since 1950 has come from additional cropland, much of it the result of colonizing new land, whereas in Africa reduction of fallow was the major influence. In Asia, already densely populated, new land was not readily available in most countries, and the increased food resulted largely from the application of technological methods pioneered in Japan, Korea and Taiwan. These methods have transformed production in many parts of Asia. In China, for example, 90 per cent of the increase since 1950 was due to higher crop yields. In India, farmers in most regions are insulated from the vagaries of the monsoon by irrigation and heavy use of fertilizers.

As a result of these advances, during the 1970s grain production – on which the poorest countries mainly depend – more than kept pace with the growth of populations, both in the world at large and in developing countries considered as a whole. Moreover it is predicted that at least until the year 2000, food output will continue to meet effective global demand, although it is now more difficult to maintain the 3 per cent a year increase in world output that was possible in the mid-1950s. However, for a number of reasons the practice of equating food resources with the number of people gives a misleading picture of the availability of food and the effects on nutrition.

First, even by the simple test which relates resources to population, many countries do not have enough food. In 1977–80 one-third of the population of the Third World lived in countries where food supplies – output, stocks and imports – were insufficient to provide the population with an adequate diet, even if distributed according to need.[4] During the 1970s, food production failed to keep pace with the growth of population in 70 countries out of a total of 126; they included countries in Eastern Europe, the Middle East and sub-Saharan Africa. The situation is particularly serious in Africa, where food output increased by only a quarter and the amount available per head declined. Of 38 countries identified by FAO's Global Information Early Warning System in 1984 as having abnormal problems, 26 were in Africa; some of them had suffered drought and poor yields for several consecutive years. There are also countries in Latin America and South Asia where output per head has fallen. Bangladesh is an extreme example: there is only a fifth of an acre per head of population and little scope for increasing the allotment.

A second reason for concern is that several countries, which by the simple test relating resouces to numbers may be said to have sufficient food, have only a small surplus and are ill-equipped to meet transitory deficiencies. These arise for a number of reasons.[5]

1 Unstable world prices. Developing countries are particularly vulnerable to instability of prices in the world market. In 1968–78 the coefficient of variation in prices ranged from about 20 per cent for maize to 35 per cent for rice. This instability was much greater than that of global production during the same period or of prices in the previous decade. The World Bank study attributed the instability on the supply side to the fact that after years of support programmes that created large grain reserves, exporters deliberately reduced stocks. This lowered the ratio of stocks to total consumption and thus caused prices to be more sensitive to fluctuations in production. But there were other influences: demand was unstable because of the sharp rise and subsequent fall in the growth of per capita income; exchange rates were volatile; domestic prices were stabilized without regard for international price fluctuations; and imports were used to offset sharp fluctuations in food production.

2 Variation in domestic production. In general, the output of the major staple foods has been unstable in developing countries, much more so than in the world market as a whole. Because of lack of foreign currency such countries have been unable to compensate for deficiencies by importing food, and few developing countries have been able to stabilize domestic food prices to the extent that has been possible in industrialized countries.

3 Variation in household purchasing power. Incomes and food production vary more for households and regions of a country than for a

[4] Grigg, D. *The World Food Problem*. Oxford, Basil Blackwell, 1985: 265.
[5] World Bank Policy Study, 1986.

country as a whole. India, for example, had relatively stable aggregate income, food production and food consumption in 1968–70; yet there was considerable instability of purchasing power from year to year in rural households.

4 Famine. This is the most severe form of transitory food insecurity and it may have several causes: wars, floods, crop failures, loss of purchasing power and high food prices. Investigation of some serious famines has shown that a reduction in the food available is not always the primary reason for famines, and attention is increasingly focussed on other causes, particularly loss of real income.[6]

A third reason, and the most serious, for the inadequacy of food to population arithmetic, is that the food available is very inequitably distributed, both between countries and between different areas and population groups of the same country. India, for example, has an overall food surplus which has more than matched the phenomenal increase of population (by a million a month: if this rate of growth continues the population will double in 20 years and India will displace China as the most populous nation). Yet for several years there has been acute famine in the north, among the eight million people who live in the arid region of Rajasthan, and deaths from starvation (for which some politicians prefer the euphemism, malnutrition) have been a source of unrest in the area of Bombay.

In relation to health, the most useful indication of inadequacy of food supply and distribution is the frequency of hunger and malnutrition. These features are not easily measured, but the World Bank study used two indices to assess the change between 1970 and 1980.

Between 340 million and 730 million people in the developing countries did not have enough income to obtain enough energy from their diet in 1980. (These estimates exclude China because data are not available). The estimate of 340 million is based on a minimum calorie standard that would prevent serious health risks and stunted growth in children. If the standard is increased to levels that allow an active working life, however, the estimate rises to 730 million. About two-thirds of the under-nourished live in South Asia and a fifth in sub-Saharan Africa. In all, four-fifths of the undernourished live in countries with very low average incomes.[7]

The study concluded that although the proportion of the population with inadequate diets declined between 1970 and 1980, because of population growth the number of people underfed probably increased. Improvement was substantial in East Asia and the Middle East, where there was rapid

[6] Sen, A. *Poverty and Famines*. Oxford, 1981.
[7] World Bank Policy Study, 1986.

economic growth, but in South Asia and sub-Saharan Africa the proportion of the population with deficient diets increased only slightly and the absolute numbers increased markedly.

Against this background it is evident that malnutrition and its sinister effects on health are common in developing countries and result mainly from international and national policies which prejudice food distribution. Most countries have enough food, and where it is deficient a relatively small increase of 5–10 per cent would eliminate malnutrition if resources were distributed equitably. The international community can contribute in many ways – with resources, with advice and not least, by refraining from encouraging or requiring Third World countries to absorb food surpluses from developed countries (the grain and butter mountains) or to adopt economic policies which contribute to their poverty. However, the causes of food insecurity are determined largely by national policies. The chief requirements are (a) to ensure an adequate food supply through policies which promote domestic production (by shifting resources from large to small farms, from industry to agriculture, from capital-intensive to labour-intensive activities) and (b) to give people who are at risk of food insecurity the opportunity to earn an adequate income. The problem of food deficiency is essentially determined by poverty.

Drinking Water and Sanitation

In the Introduction to this book I made a brief analysis of determinants of health, distinguishing basic needs (such as food and warmth) from hazards which may be either natural (from parasites) or man made (such as alcohol and atmospheric pollution). Food, the most important basic need, was discussed in relation to nutrition. We must now consider one of the most common natural hazards, the pathogens which cause diarrhoeal diseases. In certain places for limited periods other hazards may have killed more people, as in the case of plague in Europe in the fourteenth century or tobacco in some developed countries in the twentieth. But throughout the historical period, as in the Third World today, these risks were much less important than diarrhoeal diseases which killed a considerable proportion of all children within a few years of birth. In Latin America in 1978 they were responsible for about a quarter of the deaths of children under 5 years of age, and it was estimated that in 1980 they produced 4.6 million deaths (under 5 years) in developing countries (excluding China). Eighty per cent of the deaths were in children under the age of two.[8]

Because of the seriousness of diarrhoea in children, strenuous efforts are

[8] Snyder, J. D. and Merson, M. H. 'The magnitude of the global problem of acute diarrhoeal diseases: a review of active surveillance data.' *Bulletin of WHO*, 1982, **60**: 605–13.

being made to treat the diseases by oral rehydration therapy, and to reduce the frequency and severity of infection by breast feeding, good nutrition and certain vaccinations. But if health is to improve rapidly in developing countries it is also necessary to prevent transmission of the pathogens which cause diarrhoea. All major diarrhoeal pathogens are transmitted by the faecal-oral route, and the measures required for their control are improvements in water supply, in excreta disposal and in domestic and food hygiene.[9] These are the measures which led to the rapid decline of deaths from intestinal infections in industrial countries in the late nineteenth and early twentieth centuries.

Attention has been focussed internationally on the prevention of diarrhoeal diseases by the United Nations General Assembly, which designated the decade, 1981-90, as the 'International Drinking Water Supply and Sanitation Decade'. The measures with which advance is required in both urban and rural areas are now well recognized.

1 An adequate supply of clean water in or close to peoples' homes. Without this supply, water may transmit infection and personal and domestic hygiene becomes extremely difficult.
2 Hygienic disposal of excreta by ready, and preferably exclusive, access to a hygienic toilet or latrine.
3 Improvements in personal hygiene which ensure that facilities are correctly used and supported by other measures such as hand-washing, hygienic disposal of stools of young children and improved water storage (where necessary) and food hygiene.

The World Health Organization is monitoring progress during the decade and the most recent report is for the period to the end of 1983.[10] The countries providing information contain between 55 and 75 per cent of the population of developing countries (excluding China) and their data are considered to be reasonably representative of the total population of the Third World.

Prospects for rapid progress in provision of clean water and sanitation are prejudiced by a number of factors: the rapid growth of populations; a great increase in urban numbers as a result of migration from rural areas (in Africa the urban population is expected to rise by about 73 per cent in ten years); the poor state of health in many developing countries where life expectancy at birth is below 50 years, infant mortality is over 100 (per 1000 live births) and water-borne diseases are a common cause of death. In

[9] Feachem, R. G. 'Prevention better than cure.' *Diarrhoeal Diseases.* World Health Organization, April, 1986: 18-19.

[10] World Health Organization: *The International Drinking Water Supply and Sanitation Decade: Review of Regional and Global Data.* Publication No. **92**, 1986.

general, water supplies are more adequate than sanitation and both are better in urban than in rural areas. The level of services available in developing countries in 1983 was summarized as follows:

Three urban residents out of four had access to a safe water supply and about 80 per cent of them were served by a house connection.

A little over half of urban residents had access to adequate sanitation. Two rural dwellers out of five had access to a safe and adequate water supply. This is regarded as the most significant global achievement of recent years.

One rural dweller out of seven had access to appropriate sanitation. This is the service where least progress has been made and where most needs to be done. [11]

Against this background it is clear that a large increase in the rate of progress will be needed if the targets set for the decade are to be achieved. In the countries that have provided data, in urban areas an additional 184 million residents will have to be provided with water and 200 million with sanitation; in rural areas the corresponding numbers are 643 million for water and 287 million for sanitation. Moreover these increases are needed, not to provide full coverage of the populations, but to achieve the relatively low targets that have been set for 1990. In the case of rural sanitation, for example, the aim is only to increase coverage to 33 per cent of households, and even this modest advance will probably be beyond the means of some countries.

Countries were asked to give reasons for the limited progress in provision of adequate water and sanitation. The three most important constraints in all regions were lack of funds, insufficient personnel and inadequate operation and maintenance. Their relative importance varied between regions: shortage of funds was the first constraint in Africa and South Asia; in the Eastern Mediterranean it was ranked equally with inadequate water resources; in the Western Pacific it was said to be second to lack of trained staff (skilled artisans and tradesmen). However, all the major constraints are profoundly influenced by the resources available, so that the hazards attributable to inadequate water supplies and sanitation in developing countries are again due to poverty.

Control of Numbers

When assessing prospects for health in the Third World, it is important to keep in mind the significance of the timing of the major influences. In industrial countries they became effective in what was, for health and welfare, the ideal sequence. The first and most potent influence on

[11] World Health Organization.

mortality was improvement in nutrition, a consequence of a rising standard of living which preceded hygiene and other measures, in some countries by more than a hundred years. These later measures led to a further reduction of mortality, but their effect on population growth was restricted because they coincided with – indeed in France they were preceded by – a decline of the birth rate brought about by control of fertility. With expansion of food supplies and limitation of population growth an essential requirement was met, a balance between food and numbers which did not provoke Malthusian adjustment through increased mortality. Populations expanded, but at a rate more or less consistent with health needs.

In many developing countries, the time sequence of the major influences is quite different; the application of technological measures has preceded the capacity to provide sufficient food or limit numbers. In Africa, for example, before 1950 the rate of population growth was a little over 1 per cent per year and never exceeded 1.6 per cent; today the average rate is about 3 per cent. The reasons for this increase are not entirely clear, but it appears to have been due largely to the application of biomedical technology.

Many of the endemic plagues of Africa have lost their demographic impact. Smallpox has been wiped out; yellow fever is under control in many countries and, when it flares up, it is quickly contained; and malaria can be controlled or limited in its impact. Droughts and famines are not as devastating to human lives as they were in the past. Relief services, although poorly organized, do make a difference in development. All these gains can be increased manyfold with a more extensive application of the already proven intervention technologies. Thus, unlike the historical situation where economic development led the way to and accompanied population increase, in Africa populations are increasing so fast as to frustrate development efforts.[12]

Many estimates have been made of the possible consequences of the present rates of population growth. The most obvious result will be a large increase in numbers of people and it will be greatest in the poorest countries. Projections by the United Nations suggest that the world population, now about 5 billion, will be 6 billion in the year 2000, 8 billion in 2025 and 10 billion before it stabilizes in about 2100.[13]

The rates of increase are very different in different parts of the world. In Europe, North America, Japan and the Soviet Union, fertility has declined rapidly and is now at or near the level needed to maintain stable

[12] Sai, F. 'The population factor in Africa's development dilemma.' *Science*, 1984, **226**: 801–05.

[13] United Nations Department of International Economic and Social Affairs. *Long-range Global Population Projections*. Population Bulletin No. 14, 1982.

populations of about the present size. Fertility has also declined in some developing countries in Latin America and East Asia, most notably in China where there has been a spectacular fall. But elsewhere in the Third World – Africa, West Asia, South Asia and parts of Latin America – there has been no significant reduction of fertility, and populations are expected to continue to grow at about the present rates. According to medium term UN projections, before stability is achieved the population of 1980 will have increased nearly six times in Africa, about three and a half times in Latin America, and will have doubled in Asia.[14]

Another consequence of present demographic trends is the movement of people, as migrants from one country to another, but even more seriously from the point of view of health and welfare, from rural to urban areas within the same country. In 1983 there were 26 cities with populations over five million with a combined population of 252 million. It has been estimated that by the year 2000 there are likely to be 60 such cities with a combined population of 650 million; 45 of them will be in the developing world. Several of the largest cities, such as Mexico City, São Paulo and Calcutta will have over 20 million people. Moreover, the migration, formerly confined to capital cities, has begun to affect cities of secondary and even tertiary size, and many are now growing at a much faster pace. The urban migrants have already created formidable problems in respect of food, hygiene, education, housing and health; and it must be remembered that they have moved to the cities, not because they could be assured of employment, but because conditions in rural areas are very bad. 'Migrants into towns are at best underemployed and are usually unemployed, creating high crime rates in the shanty towns in which many must live. Often these septic fringes in the towns have vital statistics that are much worse than those of the rural areas.'[15]

In view of these conditions it seems remarkable that there should be doubts in some of the poorest countries about the need to restrain population growth. But the control of numbers is an emotive subject which touches on national, religious and racial sensibilities, and there are differences of opinion on whether rapid population growth should be treated as a consequence or cause of underdevelopment. Clearly it is both. Since the nineteenth century it has been evident that birth rates decline as economic conditions improve, and if resources were managed efficiently and distributed equitably between and within nations, the need to restrict numbers would probably not arise, or would not arise yet. But in the world as it exists these requirements will not be met, and limitation of numbers is an essential complement of the other measures that need to be taken –

---

[14] United Nations Department of International Economic and Social Affairs, 1982, *op. cit.*

[15] Sai, F. *Population factor.*

particularly sustained economic growth and more equitable availability of wealth. The link between health, numbers and socio-economic development is widely recognized, and few countries now question the need to lower rates of population growth. Nevertheless the setting of population targets is still a sensitive and divisive issue, and the control of numbers is not always given the attention in national planning that on health and other grounds it clearly requires.

Industrial Countries

Although many developing countries are in regions where there are special health problems from tropical diseases, their low standards of health are attributable mainly to conditions of life determined by poverty. One can be healthy in any country if one is rich; in the Third World well-to-do mothers have low maternal mortality rates and their children rarely die from diarrhoea, pneumonia and malnutrition. Moreover, the common causes of death in infancy and childhood are the same as those that were formerly predominant in temperate regions. The gross differences between health levels in developed and developing countries are therefore correctly regarded as an indication of the extent of illness that could be largely prevented by social and economic measures, above all by the relief of poverty.

But evidence of preventable illness of this kind is not confined to the Third World; there are considerable differences in health between industrial countries, and even more notably between different regions and income groups within the same country. Moreover these differences are not only in respect of diseases such as the infections which are rooted in poverty; they are also found in the chronic non-communicable diseases which have become prominent in the last few centuries. In the discussion which follows I am indebted to the *Black Report*,[16] which examined the extent and possible causes of inequalities in health observed in some developed countries of western Europe.

International Comparisons

In 1983 infant mortality rates were considerably higher in Northern Ireland, Scotland and England and Wales than in several other countries in western Europe (table 5.1). There was also variation in adult mortality rates at ages 35–44 and 45–54, but the evidence is less consistent, and some of the variation may be due to differences in ways of recording the data.

16 The Black Report. *Inequalities in Health*. London, Penguin, 1982.

Table 5.1 Infant mortality in Europe, 1983

	Deaths per 1000 live births	
	Male	Female
Northern Ireland	15.0	12.4
Scotland	12.8	9.7
France	12.3	9.0
England and Wales	11.4	9.0
Netherlands	9.3	7.5
Norway	8.7	6.9
Denmark	8.7	6.4
Sweden	7.0	7.0
Finland	6.6	5.9
Iceland	5.4	7.0

Source: United Nations Demographic Yearbook 1984. New York, United Nations (1986).

To assess the reasons for national variations in infant mortality rates the Black Report examined the frequency of different causes of death in Sweden and England and Wales in 1976 (table 5.2). The British rates were higher for all the causes examined, particularly for those – infections, acute respiratory conditions, pneumonia and accidents – which are closely associated with poverty. The differences also appeared to be related to the extent of provision of personal health services.

The Report examined the possibility that national differences were in part determined by inequalities in health within each country. It concluded that such differences exist in France, West Germany, Finland and the Netherlands, but only to a small extent in Norway and Sweden where

Table 5.2 Causes of infant mortality* in Sweden and England and Wales, 1976

	Sweden	England and Wales
Infections	0.26	0.43
Acute respiratory conditions	0.04	0.57
Pneumonia	0.13	1.02
Accidents	0.08	0.35
Various anoxic and hypoxic conditions of pregnancy	1.43	2.96
Other causes of perinatal mortality	1.07	2.30
Congenital abnormality	3.03	3.45

*Deaths per 1000 live births.
Source: The Black Report. *Inequalities in Health.* Penguin, 1982.

regional inequalities have diminished consistently over the years. Indeed one of the most impressive pieces of evidence on the causes of variation in infant mortality within and between developed countries, is the observation that differences have been virtually eliminated in five Swedish counties where formerly they were considerable (fig. 5.1). Swedish observers are also under the impression that variation in infant mortality related to family income has also been removed. Although Black and his colleagues were in no doubt that socio-economic causes were largely responsible for the observed international differences, they were unable to assess the extent to which inequalities of outcome were attributable to inequalities in provision and utilization of health services on the one hand, and to other forms of inequality on the other.

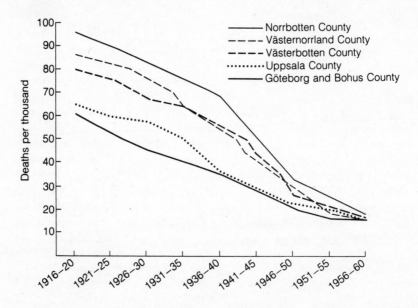

Figure 5.1   Infant mortality in five Swedish counties, 1916-60
Source: Sjolin, 'Infant mortality in Sweden' in Wallace, H. M. (ed.) *Health Care of Mothers and Children in National Health Services*, Cambridge, Mass., Ballinger, 1975.

Social Class Comparisons

Since the census of 1921 the Registrar General in England and Wales has used the occupation of the head of the family as the basis for a classification related to the standard of living. Occupations are divided into six 'social classes' according to their standing in the community, the skill they require and the income they command. Although the classification is arbitrary and takes no direct account of personal circumstances (housing, family size, education, private income) it has provided much valuable information about the association between disease and conditions of life.

Class I   Higher professional and administrative occupations (5 per cent)
Class II   Intermediate occupations (18 per cent)
Class III N   Non-manual skilled occupations (12 per cent)
Class III M   Manual skilled occupations (38 per cent)
Class IV.   Partly skilled occupations (18 per cent)
Class V   Unskilled occupations (9 per cent)

In all age groups, mortality is closely related to social class (figure 5.2). Infant mortality, particularly after the neonatal period, rises sharply with social class, so that in 1971 a child of an unskilled worker, if it survived the first four weeks of life, was five times more likely to die in the next 11 months than a child born into a professional family. A similar difference

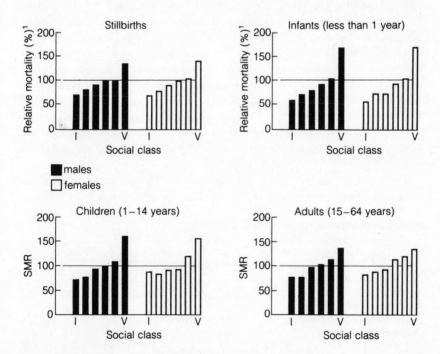

Figure 5.2 Mortality by social class and age
Source: McKeown, T. *The Role of Medicine*: 85.

existed in 1921, but infant mortality has declined in all classes and by 1971 the infant in Class V had a better chance of reaching its first birthday than an infant in Class I 40 years earlier.

Nevertheless the social class differences persist, in spite of welfare legislation (child benefits, social security, health services, assistance with housing and the like) which were thought to be of most benefit to the poor. Moreover, there was more scope for reduction of mortality from infection and other preventable causes in Class V than in Class I. Yet the percentage decline of infant mortality has been about the same for both classes, so that the proportionate decline from preventable causes has been greater in Class I.

Some causes of first year deaths show much greater social class differences than infant mortality as a whole. The death rates are many times greater for accidents and respiratory diseases in Class V than in Class I, a striking illustration of the extent to which infants die from potentially preventable and treatable conditions.

Since 1921, when social class data were first recorded, it has been evident that mortality from diseases closely related to social circumstances (tuberculosis, bronchitis, etc.) rose sharply from Class I to Class V. At that time, however, there were a few causes of death such as cardiovascular diseases and diabetes mellitus in which mortality increased from Class V to Class I. Table 5.3 shows that this relationship has now been reversed; in these, as in many other common causes of death (table 5.4) mortality is higher now for poor than for well-to-do people. There are several causes of death which show no consistent relation to social class, and the Black Report concluded that were only four in which mortality ratios are higher for Classes I and II than for IV and V: accidents to motor vehicles; malignant neoplasms of the skin; malignant neoplasm of the brain; and polyarteritis nodosa and allied conditions.

The chief conclusion which emerges is that substantial differences in health experience between poor and well-to-do people still exist in most

Table 5.3 Changes of mortality by social class*

| | Social Class | | | | | | |
	I	II	IIIN		IIIM	IV	V
Angina pectoris 1930-2	237	147		96		67	67
Acute myocardial infarction 1970-72	88	92	115		107	108	108
Diabetes mellitus 1921-23	129	149		93		75	66
1970-72	84	93	111		98	111	128

*Standardized mortality ratios, males aged 15-64, England and Wales, 1970-72.

Table 5.4 Mortality from certain causes by social class*

	Social Class					
	I	*II*	*IIIN*	*IIIM*	*IV*	*V*
Tuberculosis of respiratory system	26	41	84	89	124	254
Malignant neoplasms of stomach	50	66	79	118	125	147
Malignant neoplasms of larynx	65	65	81	102	132	194
Malignant neoplasms of bronchus, trachea and lung	53	68	84	118	123	143
Hypertensive disease	71	85	104	104	112	141
Ischaemic heart disease	88	91	114	107	108	111
Cerebrovascular disease	80	86	98	106	111	136
Ulcer of the duodenum	45	67	81	103	115	201

*Standardized mortality ratios, ages 15-64, England and Wales, 1970-72.

developed countries. The differences have persisted in respect of causes of death such as accidents and infectious diseases where they are of long standing and attributable to deficiencies and hazards rooted in poverty. But the same class differences have now appeared in mortality from non-infectious causes of sickness and death; the ill-effects of poverty on health are no longer restricted to the traditional diseases of poverty. Black and his colleagues traced the health inequalities partly to social class differences in preventive and treatment services; but they concluded that 'there is undoubtedly much that cannot be understood in terms of the impact of such specific factors. Much, we feel, can only be understood in terms of the more diffuse consequences of the class structure: poverty, work conditions (and what we termed the social division of labour) and deprivation in its various forms in the home and immediate environment, at work, in education and the upbringing of children and more generally in family and social life'.[17]

Poverty and Health

In the title of this chapter diseases due to deficiencies and hazards are referred to as diseases of poverty. This term describes accurately conditions that have prevailed during most of man's existence, and distinguishes them from others associated with the relative affluence produced by industrialization. However, this nomenclature may appear to suggest that poverty is a cause of disease, like lack of food or polluted drinking water, and that it refers to a consistent set of influences which have remained unchanged at different periods.

[17] The Black Report.

Poverty, like illiteracy and excessive numbers, is not, of course, a direct cause of disease; rather it is the main reason for the existence of many conditions that lead to disease. Inevitably these conditions have been different at different times. In the period of hunting and gathering poverty had the effects that would be expected with a primitive form of life. They changed under agriculture, and have been even more varied since industrialization. As we have noted, in the Third World and for the poor in developed countries, the traditional problems of food deficiency and unhealthy living conditions still exist. But these problems have been extended into new areas because poverty now determines the quality of many aspects of life which also profoundly affect health: education, employment, housing, transport, health services. The results are particularly significant in relation to non-communicable diseases. These diseases are largely determined by personal behaviour related to diet, tobacco, alcohol, drugs, exercise and the like, and some of them were formerly more common in well-to-do than in poor people. But the social gradient has been reversed, and remarkably it is the poor who are at greatest risk from some of the 'diseases of affluence'. Because of western influences the chronic diseases are also threatening to advance in developing countries, which are in danger of having the worst of both worlds. To the ill health to which the world has always exposed the poor, because of lack of education they are now adding the problems that they impose upon themselves.

The relation between bad health and poverty has long been obvious to sympathetic observers. Referring to conditions in France in the early nineteenth century, the doctor in Balzac's novel, *Cousin Pons*, said: 'I have spent my life seeing people die, not of their illnesses, but of that great and incurable wound, the want of money.' At the end of the century Simon, the first Chief Medical Officer in England and Wales, described poverty in its severer forms as among the worst of sanitary evils, and concluded that 'the masses will scarcely be healthy unless, to their very base, they be at least moderately prosperous'.[18]

In summary: Poverty is not a direct cause of disease, but it is the main determinant of influences that lead to disease. These influences have varied in the past according to conditions of life. In the period of hunting and gathering, the common causes of sickness and death were lack of food and environmental hazards related to the nature of the habitat. Under agriculture, food was still deficient, but there were new hazards from the infectious diseases made viable by the expanded populations and defective hygiene of urban centres.

These are still the major causes of ill health in the Third World and in the poor of technologically advanced countries. Because of inequitable

[18] Simon, J. *English Sanitary Institutions*. London, John Murray, 1897.

distribution of resources millions of people are underfed, although there is believed to be sufficient food in the world and in most countries. In many developing countries, drinking water and sanitation are grossly defective, and a considerable proportion of the deaths of children are due to diarrhoeal diseases spread by water and food. The difficulties are becoming more serious because of rapid population growth – the world's population is expected to double before it stabilizes – and the movements of people from rural to urban areas. Moreover, the long-standing health problems presented chiefly by the infections are being extended into new areas, as diseases such as diabetes, cancer and heart disease are now more common in poor than in well-to-do people, and begin to appear in developing countries under the influence of the western life style. The poor are always exposed to the worst of the prevailing conditions, and it is even more obvious today than when it was said in the nineteenth century that 'poverty in its severer forms, is among the worst of sanitary evils.'[19]

[19] *Ibid.*

Diseases of Affluence

Diseases due to Maladaptation and Hazards

A striking feature of recent health trends in developed countries is the replacement of infectious diseases that killed people early in life by non-communicable diseases that kill late in life. We have examined the influences that led to the decline of the infections, and must now consider the reasons for the predominance of non-communicable diseases. One possibility is that they were potentially present in the past, but seldom seen because most people did not live to the ages at which they are usually manifested. This explanation is consistent with an idea proposed by Haldane and examined by Medawar in his inaugural address at University College.[1] They suggested that many serious abnormalities such as cancer are genetically determined, and occur mainly at post-reproductive ages where they are largely removed from the effects of natural selection.

There is another possibility, however: the causes of death which are now common may be new diseases caused by conditions of life that have arisen during the period of industrialization. For almost the whole of his existence man lived in an environment that was relatively constant in its impact on health, and to which he was well adapted through natural selection. The expansion of populations under agriculture exposed him to new hazards which led to the predominance of the infections; but with this exception many of the determinants of health changed little before the nineteenth century. Most people still led an active outdoor life under conditions not too far removed from those of their nomadic ancestors. But with industrialization and the transfer from rural to urban life, changes have been rapid and profound, affecting not only basic influences such as food, exercise and patterns of reproduction, but also many aspects of behaviour and the environment to which people are exposed.

[1] Medawar, P. B. *The Uniqueness of the Individual*. London, Methuen, 1959: 44.

There are two lines of evidence which suggest that most non-communicable diseases are essentially new diseases: one, that although there have been large changes in living conditions since the period of hunting and gathering, there has been little change in the genetic constitution of the human population; the other, that there are good reasons for believing that the common causes of death such as cancer and heart disease are not genetic diseases established at fertilization, but are determined largely by environmental and behavioural influences.

Genetic Stability of the Human Population

In the period when conditions of life have been transformed, human genes have remained much the same. It is never possible to be certain that one has traced the origin of an idea, but so far as I am aware this seminal concept was first discussed extensively in a symposium on *The Impact of Civilisation on the Biology of Man in 1968*.[2] In his opening remarks Burnet stated that 'the average genetic constitution of present-day persons is not greatly different from what it was a hundred thousand years ago, well before the advent of any form of pastoral or agricultural activity'. The grounds for this conclusion are as follows.

Changes in gene frequency result either from mutation, which leads to the appearance of new genes, or from selection and genetic drift, which lead to redistribution of the genes that already exist. Changes in the genetic constitution of the human population by mutation are relatively slow, while changes due to selection can be quite rapid.

Man evolved slowly from near human primates over a period of a few million years, and there are no significant skeletal differences between Cro-Magnon man of 30,000 years ago and present-day man. The changes in ways of life which resulted from agriculture began about 10,000 years ago, but were substantial only 5000 years later when large cities were founded. This period of about 200 generations is much too short for major changes in genetic constitution through mutation, but the question remains whether they could have occurred through selection. Were the considerable genetic differences between the populations in different parts of the world today established during the slow evolution of *Homo sapiens*, or were they also partly due to genetic selection in the short period since the beginning of agriculture?

The evidence is not available which would permit a final answer to this question. Selection can occur very rapidly where there is substantial genetic

2 Byden, S. V. (ed.) *The Impact of Civilization on the Biology of Man*. Canberra, Australia National University Press, 1970.

variation in a population, and Haldane suggested that infectious diseases, which killed a majority of people before they could reproduce, must have had a powerful effect on evolution. The example of malaria is often cited in support of this view, for in this disease the genetic disorders of the red cell in the hereditary anaemias give a selective advantage to heterozygous carriers in response to malaria. But although the high mortalities in infancy and childhood may lead to genetically based resistance to infectious diseases, there is no evidence that other characters are significantly affected. For example, there is no reason to believe that the cycles of increasing and decreasing severity of scarlet fever, or the former high mortality from plague and gastroenteritus, have had any enduring selective effects, except possibly in relation to the diseases themselves. Most people who have considered this matter have agreed with Burnet's conclusion that 'as far as general bodily health and patterns of behaviour are concerned, one can feel reasonably confident that the genetic aspects of those qualities have not changed significantly since the days of Cro-Magnon man.' There have been minor reservations, however, in relation to food, since there may have been some genetic adaptation to changes in diet, leading, for example, to adult lactose tolerance and nitrogen thriftiness.[3]

But if reservations are needed about the possibility of genetic change since the beginning of agriculture, they are not required for the short period of industrialization, covering at most 200–300 years and 8–12 generations. In this time there can have been no significant variation in the genetic constitution of the human population, except possibly in relation to some infections. Any substantial differences in disease experience arising in this period are therefore almost certainly of environmental origin.

Changes in Conditions of Life

The implications of the conclusion that human genes have changed little during the last 100,000 years were examined in a series of papers by Boyden. He referred to what he called the principle of phylogenetic maladjustment: 'if the conditions of life of an animal deviate from those which prevailed in the environment in which the species evolved, the likelihood is that the animal will be less well suited to the new conditions than to those to which it has become genetically adapted through natural selection and consequently some signs of maladjustment may be anticipated.' This principle has a bearing on both physical and mental health,

[3] Cavalli-Sforza, L. L. 'Human evolution and nutrition.' In: Walcher, D. N. and Kretchmer, N. (eds) *Nutrition and Evolution: Food as an environmental factor in the genesis of human variability.* New York, Masson, 1981: 1-7.

being related 'not only to environmental changes of a physicochemical or material nature, such as changes in the quality of food or air, but also to various non-material environmental influences, such as certain social pressures which may affect behaviour.'[4]

Boyden discussed ways in which conditions of life have departed from those for which our hunter-gatherer genes have prepared us, and concluded that 'the majority of the disorders of which people complain in Western society are disorders of civilization, in the sense that they would have been rare or non-existent in primeval society.' This was perhaps the first clear statement of this important idea, which was later considered by others under such headings as Western diseases and diseases of affluence.

The changes which followed the introduction of agriculture were considerable; those which resulted from industrialization were profound. It is not easy to find a satisfactory classification of influences which have prejudiced health during the last two centuries, but the following are some of the important ones.

Population Growth and Urban Development

I consider these influences together because they are closely related. The new factories required labour, and as many people required work there was a rapid movement of population from country to towns. In the United Kingdom, by the middle of the nineteenth century half the population of London had been born outside the city and the proportion was even higher in Manchester, Liverpool and Glasgow.

The most obvious result of the large and dense populations and defective hygiene of cities was increased exposure to infectious diseases which are airborne or spread by the faecal-oral route. But many aspects of physical and mental health were affected by the deterioration of working and living conditions. Factories were built without regard for the health of those who worked in them, and conditions of employment were for all practical purposes uncontrolled. If we need to be reminded that our claim to progressive social policies is of recent origin, it is only necessary to recall that a hundred and fifty years ago it was possible to exploit paupers, to use female and child labour for work in mines, to force a child of six to do manual work for fourteen hours a day for six days a week, and to expose workers to the risk of industrial disease or accident without obligation to compensate them or their dependants should they fall sick or die.

The domestic environment was also bad. Back-to-back houses of poorest type were hastily erected and are still to be seen in the slum property of

[4] Boyden, S. V. 'Evolution and health.' *Ecologist*, 1973, 3: 304–09.

industrial towns. In the literature of the nineteenth century there are numerous discriptions of urban conditions, none more vivid than this account by Engels.

Passing along a rough bank, among stakes and washing lines, one penetrates into this chaos of small one-storied, one-roomed huts, in most of which there is no artificial floor; kitchen, living and sleeping-room all in one . . . Everywhere before the doors residue and offal; that any sort of pavement lay underneath could not be seen but only felt, here and there, with the feet. This whole collection of cattlesheds for human beings was surrounded on two sides by houses and a factory, and on the third by the river, and beside the narrow stair up the bank, a narrow doorway alone led out into another almost equally ill-built, ill-kept labyrinth of dwellings . . . Everything which here arouses horror and indignation is of recent origin, belongs to the industrial epoch. The couple of hundred houses, which belong to Old Manchester have been long since abandoned by their original inhabitants, the industrial epoch alone has crammed into them the swarms of workers whom they now shelter; the industrial epoch alone has built up every spot between these old houses to win a covering for the masses whom it has conjured hither from the agricultural districts and from Ireland.[5]

Dr. Johnson had said that the man who is tired of London is tired of life, but he was speaking for well-to-do people in the pre-industrial age.

In a century and a half, some of the worst features of urban conditions have been reduced or removed; but many are still to be found in the depressed city centres of developed countries, and the history is being tragically repeated in the Third World. To recognize some of the worst effects of industrialization one need only go to the centre of the old towns or to the periphery of some of the new ones.

Technological Developments

There is a wide range of hazards to be considered under the heading of technological developments. They could be classified according to the nature of their sources – mechanical, chemical, electrical, nuclear – but in relation to health it will be convenient to consider briefly some of the effects.

Before the eighteenth century nearly everyone had access to clear air; it was reported recently that even in Switzerland one must now go above 6000 feet to find it. The pollution of air and water results from the discharge of domestic and industrial effluents. The main sources of atmospheric pollution are the combustion of solid fuel (coal and coke) and

[5] Engels, F. *The Condition of the Working Class in England in 1844.* London, George Allen and Unwin Ltd., 1892.

of petroleum products (kerosene, diesel oil and motor spirit). The use of nuclear power does not cause atmospheric pollution, but it leads to the discharge of waste products into the sea and introduces hazards from radiation and from the possibility of an occasional major disaster such as from the nuclear reactor at Chernobyl near Kiev in 1987.

Hazards arise from mechanized transport of all kinds – by sea, air and land – but the most common risks are undoubtedly from traffic accidents. Some risks from technological developments are decreasing, usually because of improved methods and stricter controls (as in the case of coal mining); but with continuous pressure to make and sell automobiles, risks from traffic are likely to increase. Indeed, there must be many people, alarmed by traffic and disenchanted by television, who sympathize with W. H. Auden's view that the most pernicious consequences of the Industrial Revolution were the inventions of the camera and the combustion engine.

There has been a large increase in the use of chemicals in agriculture and in food. Chemical fertilisers were introduced in the mid nineteenth century and pesticides a little later; their use has increased rapidly in recent years, 10 and 33 times respectively in developing countries (chapter 5). They have contributed greatly to food production, and on balance have done more good than harm; but where more expensive methods can be afforded it has been thought right to avoid the risks by use of organic farming methods, essentially a return to traditional practices which do not depend on chemicals. Similar considerations have led to concern about food additives, which are used for many purposes related to the production, preservation and promotion of sales of food.

Diet

The most significant changes related to health since industrialization were probably in respect of food. I have suggested that the increase in food consumption and the reduction of infection conveyed (particularly by milk) were major reasons for the decline of deaths from infectious diseases; until the nineteenth century the amount of food was far more important than its composition. (Chamfort said that the population was divided into two classes, those with appetites but no dinners and those with dinners but no appetites.) In the present context, however, we are concerned with the health consequences of changes in the composition of the diet.

Foods consumed today can be divided into four basic groups: meat and fish; vegetables and fruit; milk and milk products; and bread and cereals. Hunter-gatherers had few cereal grains and no dairy products; under agriculture cereals became the predominant food and milk and its products were irregularly available, generally in short supply.

Against this background it is easy to see the extent to which we have departed from the kind of diet for which our genes have prepared us. In the light of present knowledge, the most significant changes are the removal of fibre and the increased consumption of fat, sugar and salt. It is possible to date these changes with reasonable accuracy.

Braudel tells us that the revolution in the making of bread occurred between 1750 and 1850. The practice of sifting flour to remove the bran was practised from the fourteenth century or earlier in France; but white bread was a rarity and a luxury, eaten by only about 4 per cent of the European population. From the middle of the eighteenth century, however, wheat gradually replaced other cereals in many countries, and bread was increasingly made from flour that had the bran removed. Nevertheless the change in bread making occurred slowly, and it was only from about 1850 that most people in Europe had white bread. To the extent that lack of fibre contributes to the occurrence of digestive and other diseases, it has been a common influence for a little more than a hundred years.

In relation to health, probably the most important change in diet was increased consumption of fat, derived chiefly from dairy products. They were not taken in the vegetarian Far East, and although milk, eggs and cheese were eaten in some European countries, because of difficulties in production and preservation, consumption was limited. We can date the increase in the amount of fat mainly to the widespread use of dairy products from the beginning of the present century, when refrigeration and pasteurization made it possible to handle milk and its products safely.

Sugar is an ancient food, and was in use in India and China in the eighth century. But its extensive production began in Brazil in the sixteenth century, and from that time it was taken as a food rather than as a medicine. Nevertheless, for some time it remained a luxury, and until the eighteenth century there were large areas of Europe where it was unknown.[6] Its widespread use is therefore quite recent, and consumption at present high levels has occurred only in this century, greatly advanced by the promotion of refined sugar and processed foods.

For centuries there has been a world-wide trade in salt, which was essential for the preservation of meat and fish. But it had numerous other uses, in preservation of fats and vegetables (from the eighteenth century) and to make food more palatable to those who had acquired a taste for salt, a feature of both the European and the Eastern cooking traditions. It is said that in Europe about 20 gms per person was consumed daily,[7] so that considerable amounts of salt have been taken by some people for quite a

[6] Braudel, F. *The Structure of Everyday Life*. London, Fontana Press, 1985.
[7] *Ibid.*

long time, although others, more deprived or perhaps more fortunate, have had little or none.

To summarize these conclusions concerning diet: changes in composition have occurred quite recently and the times and extent of their introduction have varied between different populations. Restricting attention to developed countries, at the levels which would affect the diets of most people, the reduction of fibre and addition of salt probably occurred during the nineteenth century, and the consumption of large amounts of fat and sugar from about the beginning of the twentieth. All these changes are significant departures from the diets of hunter-gatherers whose genes we have inherited, but the largest, and probably the most important change, was the increase in the amount of fat which followed discovery of methods of sterilizing and preserving dairy products.

Pattern of Reproduction

The major change which can be dated most accurately is in the pattern of reproduction, for it is reflected sensitively by the behaviour of the birth rate. I have given reasons for believing that although there were earlier variations in fertility, they were small in comparison to those which have occurred in the last two centuries, the period of the modern rise of population. Fortunately, in some developed countries birth and death rates have been recorded nationally for most of this period. The birth rate declined sharply in France from 1800, in Sweden, Ireland and England and Wales from the 1870s and in most other developed countries about the same time or a little later.

The changes in reproduction which are known or can be inferred from the decline of the birth rate are very large: they include later ages for its beginning and end, fewer births, longer intervals between births and less frequent breast feeding. Although possibly unrelated to the birth rate, there has also been a reduction of the age of the menarche and an advance in the age of the menopause. No doubt there have been other less obvious changes, for example associated with the general increase in body stature and weight, and from loss of weight, as in anorexia nervosa. It has not yet been possible to establish a clear relation between these changes and diseases of the reproductive system, but this may be due to the difficulties which beset the investigations. Unfortunately nineteenth-century records do not enable us to see whether deaths from breast cancer increased after the change in the pattern of reproduction, in the way that twentieth century statistics of cause of death show the temporal relation between lung cancer and smoking.

Tobacco and Alcohol

In three important respects the history of tobacco and alcohol is analogous to that of the dietary constituents that we have just considered: they were probably unavailable or rarely available in the period when our genes were fashioned; they have been taken to a variable extent for centuries; their widespread public use is recent, in the present century in the case of tobacco.

It is hardly possible to exaggerate the significance of tobacco, not only as a cause of disease, but also as unequivocal evidence of the relation between conditions of life and the occurrence of non-communicable diseases. In many diseases there are multiple influences whose effects are difficult to dissociate from one another, and this may account for the reluctance of some medical scientists to attach much importance to lifestyle as a cause of disease. But they recognize tobacco as an exception, because the effects are so large and clear-cut that they appear even in small surveys. Indeed the link between smoking and cancer of the lung meets epidemiological requirements which might be regarded as analogous to the postulates that Koch outlined for the study of infections.

1 There is an epidemic of the disease.
2 A plausible agent (smoking) is associated with the disease.
3 The use of the agent has increased, and the increase is in the expected temporal relation to the epidemic (in both sexes).
4 Removal of the agent has lowered mortality from the disease in doctors and others.

In many non-communicable diseases these requirements are difficult to meet, but the relation between alcohol and cirrhosis of the liver is so striking that there is no doubt about its importance as a cause of the disease.

Physical Exercise

There is also little doubt about the time when the physical demands of life were greatly reduced. At all times there were people, in what would have been regarded as privileged positions, who limited their movements, generally by relying on others to do their work for them. In both urban and rural life physical demands were reduced by mechanization from the eighteenth century, but the widespread reduction has resulted from the introduction of the automobile since 1900. Indeed the effects of the car on physical condition and of television on literacy are perhaps the chief justifications for Auden's condemnation of the combustion engine and the camera, referred to above.

Illicit Drugs

What are now regarded as illicit drugs have been available since ancient times, but there has undoubtedly been a large increase in their production and distribution in the last three centuries. Opium, for example, was often consumed in the West, particularly in Turkey, and in the East it spread from India to China and the East Indies. According to Braudel, 'the great turning point came about 1765, just after the conquest of Bengal, when a monopoly of poppy fields was established to the advantage of the East India Company.'[8] There has been an even greater increase in the present century, and illicit drugs are now produced and distributed widely throughout the world.

Evidence that Non-Communicable Diseases are New Diseases

In the discussion to this point we have concluded that human genes were unchanged during the short period of industrialization when conditions of life changed greatly, and that this is likely to have led to both physical and mental disorders. We must now consider more direct evidence which suggests that this is the best explanation for the predominance of non-communicable diseases as causes of sickness and death.

1 Experience of other animals. The diseases are rare or absent in the other animals most closely related to man. As noted in chapter 1, cancer and heart disease are sometimes found in primates kept in the artificial conditions of zoos and laboratories, but they are very uncommon in wild animals in their natural habitats where they are not in contact with the man-made environment.

2 Twin evidence. The so called common diseases are not determined at fertilization by single-gene defects or chromosomal aberrations, and they are usually attributed to the interaction between multiple genetic and environmental influences. However, their conditions vary between diseases and for the same disease in different environments, so that we need to be extremely cautious when attempting to assess, particularly in quantitative terms, the effects of heredity and environment in the causation of human disease.

Twin studies have been used extensively for this purpose. The only individuals with identical genes are monozygotic twins, and observed differences in their disease experience can usually be attributed to their prenatal or postnatal environments. (Even about this conclusion there must

[8] *Ibid.*

be a reservation: Edwards has noted that 'differences between similar cells in similar tissues must be largely fortuitous and it would be wrong to infer that, because identical twins show little similarity in their liability to some diseases, particularly such focal diseases as neoplasia, environmental features must therefore be important'.)[9] However, the matter is usually considered the other way round: if identical twins are consistently both affected in different environments, the abnormality is said to be determined by their common genes. The usual procedure is to identify pairs in which one twin is affected, and inquire how frequently the other twin has the same condition (is concordant). The results are then compared with those of dizygotic twins and sometimes other relatives. In no common disease is concordance 100 per cent; but when it is consistently high in twins exposed to different environments, say over 80 per cent and at least twice the rate in non-identical twins, it seems permissible to conclude that the condition is largely determined by genes of high specificity.

In the non-communicable diseases which are the leading causes of death in developed countries these requirements are not met; concordance rates are quite low and not much higher for monozygotic than for dizygotic pairs. That is to say, the frequency with which two children of the same family are both affected is not much greater if they are genetically identical than if they are not.

In their review of twin evidence, Hrubec and Robinette stated that 'monozygotic concordances for cancer at all sites and for specific cancers at the more common sites are low, as are the estimates of heritability of the liability for these diseases'.[10] They concluded that genetic and early environmental factors shared by twins explain very little of the cause of most cancers.

The evidence related to coronary heart disease is less consistent, but again concordance rates are low and not very different from monozygotic and dizygotic pairs. In a Danish study the rates were 0.39 for monozygotic and 0.26 for dizygotic male twins, and 0.44 and 0.14 respectively for female twins.[11] The results appear to vary considerably in relation to diagnostic criteria and environmental influences such as physical activity and stress. In diabetes, concordance rates in monozygotic pairs are said to be higher in the adult onset type than in the juvenile form of the disease.

3 Secular trends. There have been some remarkable changes in the incidence of some non-communicable diseases in genetically stable

[9] Edwards, J. H. 'The genetic basis of common disease.' *Am. J. Med.*, 1963, **34**: 631.

[10] Hrubec, Z. and Robinette, C. D. 'The study of human twins in medical research.' *N. Engl. J. Med.*, 1984, **310**, 435–41.

[11] Harvald, B. and Hauge, M. 'Coronary occlusion in twins.' *Acta. Genet. Med. Gemellol (Roma)*, 1970, **19**: 248–50.

populations. On the basis of data from 28 mainly industrialized countries, the World Health Organization reported that from 1960 to 1980 male deaths from cancer (all types) increased by 55 per cent, or 40 per cent when a correction is made for the increasing age of the populations. In the same period mortality from cancer of the lung (age corrected) increased by 78 per cent for males and 80 per cent for females. There was also an increase in breast cancer (by 43 per cent), and indeed in all the other types examined with the exception of cervical and stomach cancers, which showed relatively small but consistent decreases.[12] This change is particularly significant in Japan, where stomach cancer is the most common form of the disease. In recognition of the environmental and behavioural origins of cancer, and of the appearance of those influences in the Third World, the World Health Organization predicted that 'there will be an epidemic of cancer in the majority of the developing world by the year 2000'. In this context we should also note the remarkable differences in disease death rates in different countries. For example, age-adjusted death rates of breast and colon cancer in many parts of the world are less than one fifth of the rates in the United States. Willett and MacMahon concluded that these differences cannot be accounted for by variation in genetic predisposition.[13]

The influence of smoking on cancer mortality is so large that the rise in deaths was predictable; the recent decline of mortality from coronary heart disease in the United States and several other countries was more surprising. In the United States it affected both sexes, both major racial groups and all three adult decades. A reduction of deaths has also occurred in Finland. It is not yet clear how much of the change was due to each of the influences that may have been involved – treatment, reduction of blood pressure and blood cholesterol and changes in lifestyle, particularly in relation to diet and exercise. What is obvious is that the change was due to such influences, rather than to variation in genetic predisposition.

4 Change of environment. A racial group which has changed its environment and associated ways of life exhibits the disease pattern of the population with which it shares its environment rather than that of the population with which it shares its genes. This experience has been particularly striking in cancer, whose frequency differs widely by type and country. Japanese migrants in Hawaii, for example, had the high stomach cancer rates seen in Japan, but the rates had fallen in their children. There was a sharp increase in the risk of breast cancer for Japanese women living

[12] World Health Organization. *Weekly Epidemiological Record*, 1985, **60**, No. 17.

[13] Willett, W. C. and MacMahon, B. 'Diet and cancer – an overview.' *N. Engl. J. Med.* 1984, **310**: 633–8; 697–703.

[14] Haenszel, W., Kurihara, M., Segi, M. and Lee, R. K. C. 'Stomach cancer among Japanese in Hawaii.' *JNCI*, 1972, **49**: 969–88.

in the San Francisco Bay Area.[15] For cancers of the stomach, intestinal tract and lung, rates for Polish migrants to the United Kingdom were intermediate between the levels of people living in Poland and England and Wales.[16]

5 'Western diseases'. Perhaps the most persuasive evidence that the non-communicable diseases are essentially new is the observation that they are rare in populations which have retained their traditional way of life, but begin to appear when they change to the western lifestyle. In *Western Diseases* Trowell and Burkitt brought together reports by 34 contributors who described their experience of changes in the pattern of disease in several countries as westernization occurs.[17] There are four main lines of evidence, not all equally secure. (a) Until recently many of the non-communicable diseases now predominant in the West were uncommon or absent in hunter-gatherers and peasant agriculturalists. (b) When these populations change from their traditional ways of life to those of developed countries, they begin to exhibit the western pattern of disease. (c) The incidence of some of the diseases has declined in western populations which have reversed certain features of their lifestyle to bring it closer to that of peasant agriculturalists. (d) Of the multiple influences responsible for the western pattern of disease, Trowell and Burkitt considered that dietary changes are probably the most important.

The evidence assembled on the first two points is impressive. Before 1940, in Africans of Kenya and Uganda, blood pressure did not rise with age and essential hypertension was rarely seen; it is now a common disease. Obesity was almost unknown in 1930, when Julian Huxley noted with amazement that 'almost the only fat woman I saw in Africa' worked in the Nairobi brewery; today 'the towns of East Africa contain many fat upper class Africans and their leaders seen on television are often grossly obese'. (Trowell suggested that obesity and the associated diabetes probably emerged as common disorders in the English upper classes in the late eighteenth century, when sugar was first reported in their urine). In Kenya in the 1930s, diabetes was rare in Africans but not in Europeans and Indians; there are now large diabetic clinics in all town hospitals. Cerebrovascular disease was the first arterial disease of clinical significance to emerge in Africans. Before 1948 a case due to hypertension was rarely or never seen; in 1970 it was the commonest cause of death in a large series of neurological

[15] Buell, P. 'Changing incidence of breast cancer in Japanese-American women.' *JNCI*, 1973, **51**: 1479–83.

[16] Adelstein, A. M., Staszewski, J. and Muir, C. S. 'Cancer mortality in 1970–1972 among Polish-born migrants in England and Wales.' *Br. J. Cancer*, 1979, **40**: 464–75.

[17] Trowell, H. C. and Burkitt, D. P. (eds) *Western Diseases: Their Emergence and Prevention.* London, Edward Arnold, 1981.

patients in a Ugandan hospital. Coronary artery disease is the last major cardiovascular western disease to appear – the first clinical reports of cases were made quite recently in Uganda (1956) and in Kenya and Tanzania (1968). And it is said that 'coronary thrombosis has begun only recently to emerge in Zimbabwe Africans and angina remains a rare disease'.

On the basis of observations of this kind from many parts of the world, Trowell and Burkitt prepared a provisional list of Western diseases. In addition to those already mentioned, it includes gallstones, varicose veins, constipation, appendicitis, diverticular disease, haemorrhoids, cancers of the bowel, chest and lung and dental caries. While there may be differences of opinion about the acceptabilty of some of the conditions as Western diseases, the general conclusion that they are appearing in developing countries where formerly they were rare is not in doubt.

Maladaptation and Affluence

In the preceding discussion non-communicable diseases were attributed to maladaptation and to hazards which have arisen in the last few centuries, and in the title of this chapter these influences were equated with affluence. As a description of the major changes which have occurred the terms are reasonably satisfactory, but they may lead to misunderstanding on one or two points and it will be desirable to say a little more about them.

We have examined reasons for believing that the predominance of non-communicable diseases resulted from conditions of life established since industrialization. These conditions differed greatly from those that prevailed under agriculture, and still more from conditions in the period of hunting and gathering in relation to which our genes evolved. It therefore seems justified to attribute the present disease pattern largely to maladaptation, to exposure to conditions for which we are genetically ill-equipped. It is of course conceivable that human genes could adapt to some of the changes – in diet, exercise, smoking, reproduction and the like – as the genes of our ape-like ancestors adjusted in the remote past to life on the plains. But adaptation would take a very long time, and it will not occur at all if natural selection is checked by medical or other interventions. If we are to breed a race fit to smoke we must allow plenty of time, and we must encourage children to light up at an early age, so that they have a reasonable chance of killing themselves before they can reproduce.

But not all the hazards that have resulted from industrialization are due to maladaptation. Whatever their genes, men and women could be damaged or killed by road traffic, pesticides, adverse working conditions, ionizing radiation, atmospheric pollution and the like. It is therefore necessary to attribute the non-communicable diseases not only to mal-adaptation, but also to a wide range of hazards that have appeared in the last two centuries.

In one sense it seems reasonable to regard the maladaptation and hazard as a consequence of the relative affluence which was a by-product of industrialization; sedentary living and excessive food consumption are clearly made possible by resources in excess of essential requirements. But there are other hazards such as pesticides and atmospheric pollution which are only indirectly due to affluence; and the use of the term seems anomalous when applied to influences such as smoking and drug addiction which are becoming more common in poor than in well-to-do people. Nevertheless for the reasons discussed in the introduction to Part II, I have used the term 'diseases of affluence' because it is less objectionable than the obvious alternatives, and because it contrasts with 'diseases of poverty' which describes accurately the conditions that have prevailed for almost the whole of human existence.

In summary: Several lines of evidence indicate that the non-communicable diseases now common in developed countries are new diseases, caused by conditions that have arisen in the last few centuries. First, there has been little change in the genetic constitution of the human population in the last 100,000 years and none in the last 200 years, so that our genes have prepared us for ways of life very different from those of today. Second, living conditions have changed profoundly since industrialization, in ways that might be expected to prejudice both physical and mental health: increased size and density of populations; transfer from rural to urban life; reduction of fibre and increase of fat, sugar and salt in the diet; increased use of tobacco, alcohol and illicit drugs; reduction of physical exercise; changes in the pattern of reproduction, with fewer and later pregnancies. Most of these changes are relatively recent, and some – smoking, reduction of exercise and excessive consumption of fat and sugar – have occurred on a large scale only in this century.

More direct evidence that the non-communicable diseases are new is provided by observations on the common causes of deaths, such as cancer, cardiovascular disease and diabetes. (a) The incidence of some of the diseases has varied widely in genetically stable populations. (b) A racial group which has changed its environment and associated ways of life exhibits the disease pattern of the population with which it shares its environment rather than that of the population with which it shares its genes. (c) The frequency with which two children of the same family are affected is not much greater if they are genetically identical than if they are not. (d) The diseases are uncommon or absent in hunter-gatherers and peasant agriculturalists, but begin to appear when they change from their traditional ways of life to the Western lifestyle.

I conclude that most non-communicable diseases have arisen from exposure to conditions of life for which we are genetically ill-equipped, but some, such as accidents and industrial diseases are caused by hazards to which genetic adaptation is hardly conceivable. The diseases can therefore be said to be due to maladaptation and to certain hazards which have emerged in the industrial period.

PART III

Disease Control

Introduction

In the light of the preceding analysis of disease origins, basic requirements for health can be summarized as follows. In the Third World, health depends in large part on removal of the long-standing deficiencies and hazards associated with poverty, without incurring the new risks that have appeared under modern conditions, partly as a by-product of affluence. In industrialized countries, the chief requirements are to control for health purposes an environment which is largely man's creation, and to modify those features of behaviour for which the genes are ill-adapted. In both developed and developing countries, the formidable problems determined before birth present a continuing challenge to medical research and health services. But this is no more than a preliminary appraisal, and it will be necessary to examine more closely the possibilities in each of the disease classes in the chapters which follow.

Before proceeding with this enquiry, however, I should clarify the interpretation of disease control. In the sense in which I am using the term, a disease can be said to be controlled when it is prevented or cured, and the analysis of disease origins in Part II was designed to facilitate an examination of different methods. In theory, genetic diseases determined at fertilization might be controlled by replacement of defective genes, by avoidance of the conception or birth of those likely or certain to be affected, or by successful treatment; diseases not determined at fertilization might be controlled by removal of the environmental or behavioural influences which lead to them, by increasing the body's resistance to disease (for example, by immunization or improved nutrition), or again by successful treatment. It will be evident that when interpreted in this way, disease control is concerned with the complete solution of health problems, and only indirectly with the task on which western medical research and practice are largely engaged, the treatment and care of the sick.

It need hardly be said that the focus on the prevention or cure of disease is in no sense a criticism of the enormous importance attached to the care of the sick. Even if preventive measures were as comprehensive as we would like them to be, and so successful that we rarely encountered disease or disability attributable to a hazardous environment or the twin threats of poverty and affluence, there would remain the formidable problems of illness determined before birth or associated with the end of life. The care of the sick is, and will remain, the central medical task, requiring large resources and the attention of most doctors. But health services, broadly conceived, should be concentrated where they can be most effective. Whether resources should in some circumstances be transferred from treatment of disease to more effective preventive measures is an important question, but it is outside the scope of the present discussion of disease control.

The main purpose of the analysis of disease origins was to clarify, and in a sense simplify, our understanding of the ways in which diseases arise. There are several reasons for misunderstanding in the past, particularly the failure to distinguish genetic diseases from those which arise after fertilization, and to recognize that as human genes have changed little since the Pleistocene, disease experience is determined essentially by conditions of life. This is true of both infections and non-communicable diseases.

The question will inevitably be asked whether on the basis of a preliminary analysis of disease origins it is possible to make an adequate assessment of the most promising methods of future disease control. The answer, of course, is that it is not. The classification of diseases according to their origins should be regarded rather as a contribution to the changing medical paradigm (to use Thomas Kuhn's terminology), which will lead to new ideas about the nature and management of disease problems. Nevertheless, it seems desirable to give some indication of the kinds of control which are suggested by the examination of origins, and this is the purpose of Part III.

Finally, something should be said about the timescale on which the proposals are based. In general, they are concerned with the short and medium term, that is with developments which are possible or likely on the basis of present knowledge or foreseeable extensions of it. This approach does not of course overlook the probability that in time there will be new discoveries which will greatly improve the prospects for disease control. Nevertheless we should recognize that a great deal of the knowledge required for rapid improvement in health is already available, and what is needed for achievement of an acceptable standard of health throughout the world is not so much new basic knowledge as effective managerial procedures and political will.

7

Prenatal Diseases

In chapter 4, genetic disorders established at fertilization were considered separately from malformations and other congenital conditions determined later in uterine life. The same distinction is even more necessary in discussion of prenatal disease control, since diseases established at fertilization can be managed only by avoidance of conception, abortion or treatment, whereas those that arise later offer the possibility of prevention by modification of environmental and behavioural influences.

Abnormalities Determined at Fertilization

If we exclude disorders manifested after birth, usually late in life, genetic diseases occur in about one in a hundred births. In principle they can be managed in three ways: by prevention of conception; by elimination during pregnancy; and by treatment. It will be convenient to consider these possibilities in order of their increasing feasibility.

Treatment

It is well recognized that on the basis of present knowledge treatment is the least promising of the three approaches. In an extensive review of the application of genetics to clinical practice, Weatherall concluded that 'for the vast majority of genetic disorders there is no form of treatment other than symptomatic therapy.'[1] The exceptions to which he refers include replacement therapy for the missing coagulation factor in haemophilia, long-term transfusion therapy for thalassaemia, replacement with immuno-globulin for children with inherited forms of hypogammaglobulinae-mia, and diets which prevent accumulation of toxic metabolites, as in

[1] Weatherall, D. J. *The New Genetics and Clinical Practice*. London, Nuffield Provincial Hospitals Trust. 1982: 90-9.

phenylketonuria. Most of these treatments are costly, traumatic for the patient and give results which are often unsatisfactory; indeed in some cases they could be said to increase the difficulties. The problems are well illustrated by treatment of children with thalassaemia, who develop normally with regular blood transfusions, only to die in the second or third decade as a result of iron loading from transfused blood. It is easier to bear an absence than a parting, and there can be few partings more heart-rending than the prolonged leave-taking between parents and a child whose early death is inevitable, but who has lived long enough to wreathe a flowery band to bind it to the earth. The medical scientist who discovers treatment which leads to this result is in some ways in the position of a nuclear physicist whose work has led to development of weapons which he regrets but is unable to reverse.

Results from attempts to replace missing enzymes in metabolic disorders have also been disappointing. The correction of genetic blood diseases by bone-marrow transplantation is not very successful, but it is still at an early stage and Weatherall considers it may have a place in the treatment of crippling disorders such as chronic granulomatous disease.[2]

Inevitably the lack of success of most forms of treatment has turned attention to the possibilities of gene replacement therapy, which would be 'the ultimate achievement in the application of genetic engineering technology to human disease.'[3] To succeed, this approach must meet at least three requirements: a new gene must be put into the appropriate target cell and must remain in it, the new gene must be regulated appropriately; and the new gene must not harm a cell. Perutz has assessed the formidable difficulties which arise in meeting these requirements.

The collection of chromosomes that carry human genes consists of a meter of DNA distributed over forty-six chromosomes, and its information content is equivalent to a library of five thousand volumes. To cure a genetic disease, the genetic engineer has to find and correct what may be no more than a single misprint in any one of these volumes. Techniques for finding misprints are very advanced, but those for correcting them are haphazard. Genetically defective strains of mice can be transformed into healthy strains only by injecting thousands of copies of DNA containing the healthy gene into the fertilized eggs. The hope is that at least one of these copies will be incorporated into the chromosomes in such a way as to cure the defect.

This haphazard way may succeed in some subjects, but in others the injected gene may be exposed in the wrong tissue at the wrong time or its accidental insertion into another gene may cause a new genetic defect. This does not matter too much in experiments with mice, where scientists can select the healthy mouse among many

2 *Ibid.*
3 *Ibid.*

defective ones, but it would be unacceptable for human beings. To correct a genetic lesion reliably, a healthy gene would have to be spliced in the correct position in place of the defective one. There are no techniques in sight for doing this.[4]

In the light of this analysis of the problems it is difficult to disagree with the conclusion that 'we are a long way from the stage when the insertion of genes into human cells can be seriously contemplated.'[5] The results of treatment by other means are so poor that attention is inevitably turned to other approaches.

Prevention of Conception

Most people would probably agree that the ideal solution of the problems presented by serious genetic disorders would be to avoid their conception. This approach does not raise the formidable difficulties associated with treatment, and it sidesteps most of the awkward ethical issues which make antenatal diagnosis followed by abortion repugnant to some people.

Nevertheless the primary prevention of genetic disorders has its own difficulties. To succeed it would be necessary to identify people who would be likely to have affected children, and to persuade them not to marry or, if married, not to reproduce.

By avoidance of reproduction of affected persons it would be possible to eliminate dominant genotypes which are completely manifested before reproductive age. This requirement is met by only a few rare abnormalities, for example, by achondroplasia and a certain type of juvenile cataract. In most dominant genotypes the abnormality is not completely manifested in all environments, or it does not appear until after reproduction has begun. Huntington's chorea is an example of a condition due to a dominant gene which cannot be eliminated in this way, because it becomes evident only in middle life when those affected may have reproduced.

Most single genes which cause genetic disorders are recessive and are manifested only in the homozygous state. The number of individuals who carry the gene but are not themselves affected (the heterozygotes) is much larger than the number of affected (the homozygotes). For example, only about 1 in 20,000 people exhibit albinism (are homozygous), whereas 1 in 70 carry the gene but are not affected. Hence only a small proportion of those affected have affected parents, the suppression of whose reproduction would have little effect on the frequency of the gene. Reduction of the incidence of a sex-linked recessive condition, such as haemophilia, would

[4] Perutz, M. F. 'Brave new world.' *New York Review of Books*. 1985, XXXII, No. 14: 17.
[5] Weatherall, D. J. *The New Genetics*: 60–89.

be more feasible, but it would require restriction of reproduction of daughters and sisters of affected males, as well as of the affected males themselves.

It is evident that, to be effective, primary prevention of genetic disorders could not be restricted to families with affected members, but would need to be extended to the general population in order to discover heterozygotes. Tests are available for the presence of many of the abnormalities, although there are none for some single-gene defects such as cystic fibrosis and Huntington's chorea.

The most promising application of primary prevention would appear to be in common conditions which can be readily detected. These requirements are well met by the hereditary anaemias, which reach high frequencies in certain populations and in which heterozygous carriers can be identified by relatively simple and cheap tests. It is therefore disappointing that an attempt to apply this method was judged to be a complete failure, and Weatherall concluded that the effectiveness of primary prevention by screening and genetic counselling is uncertain.[6] The basic difficulties which beset this approach are (a) the lack of reliable tests, (b) the difficulty of applying tests to the general population, and (c) the preference of parents who may have affected children for pregnancy followed, if necessary, by abortion.

Antenatal Diagnosis Followed by Abortion

We may appear to have been led to serious consideration of the third approach to control of genetic disorders by the limitations of the other two; but secondary prevention by antenatal screening is more than a last resort. Even when parents likely to have an affected child are known – either because they are carriers of a defective gene or because they have previously had an abnormal birth – they may still wish to face the risks of pregnancy, particularly if an abnormal fetus can be identified and removed.

Antenatal screening is most widely, and perhaps most happily, used for discovery of conditions which can be treated effectively, as in the case of rhesus haemolytic disease. But as most genetic abnormalities cannot be treated satisfactorily they are identified during pregnancy so that an affected fetus can be removed by abortion.

Large-scale screening of pregnancies obviously cannot be used if the genetic abnormality cannot be identified, and it is inefficient with disorders which occur at low frequency. But it is quite feasible where a recognizable

6 *Ibid.*: 100–26.

defect is common, as is Tay-Sachs disease in some Jewish people and the haemoglobinaemias in many populations.

The use of antenatal screening is well illustrated by B thalassaemia. Parents likely to have an affected child can be identified, and if pregnancy occurs the risks to the fetus are known. The abnormality can be discovered in the fetus, either by fetal DNA analysis or by fetal blood sampling and globin chain synthesis a few weeks later. By these methods the number of children born with B thalassaemia was reduced from 70 to 2 in Cyprus, from 300 to 150 in Greece and from 70 to 30 in Sardinia. The same approach is now being used in other populations where the defect is common.[7]

In view of the poor prospects of gene replacement, primary prevention and treatment of genetic disorders, secondary prevention through antenatal screening is likely to remain the chief resource in the foreseeable future. The difficulties associated with the approach are broadly of three kinds: scientific problems, particularly lack of knowledge of the aetiology and natural history of the diseases, and inadequate methods of recognition of affected children and of parents who are carriers; managerial and economic problems, which are very serious in developing countries in view of lack of trained staff and finance; and ethical issues, in populations which object on religious or other grounds to the use of abortion.

Abnormalities Determined After Fertilization

Congenital Malformations

It is a sobering thought that after several decades of research, a number of international conferences and many other meetings, seminars and symposia, the problem of human malformations remains essentially unchanged. A causative agent – thalidomide – has been discovered and withdrawn; an infection, rubella, is so often teratogenic that when recognized in pregnant women it is accepted as grounds for abortion; some malformations can be identified and removed during pregnancy, and a few which formerly were lethal or disabling, particularly those of the heart, can now be treated successfully. In spite of these and some other less striking advances, the level of infant deaths due to malformations – a useful index of their frequency – has remained about the same, and with the decline of other causes of death their relative contribution to infant mortality in developed countries has increased. Between 1940 and 1964 the proportion of still-

[7] *Ibid.*: 100–26.

births and infant deaths attributed to malformations in Scotland rose from one in ten to nearly one in four.

The problems presented by malformations can be discussed conveniently at three stages: before conception; during pregnancy; and as they present from birth.

Before conception The most satisfactory solution, if attainable, would be avoidance of pregnancy in women whose children are likely to be affected. Unfortunately, on the basis of present knowledge the parents of such children cannot often be identified. It might seem possible to reduce the prevalance of malformations by discouraging further reproduction of parents who have had a malformed child. However, many parents are prepared to take the risk of recurrence; indeed when a malformed child dies within a year of birth, the interval before the next pregnancy is somewhat shorter than for the general population of mothers. Moreover, even if there were no further pregnancies of parents who have had one malformed birth, the effect on the frequency of malformations would not be large. This is merely another way of saying that in most sibships there is only one affected child.

Yet another possibility is avoidance of pregnancy in circumstances where a malformation is likely to occur, and epidemiologists have given much attention to influences such as maternal age, birth order, season of birth and social class. However, except in Down's syndrome the effect of these influences is slight.

During pregnancy The control of malformations during pregnancy can be considered either by the removal or (in the case of infections) modification of teratogenic agents, or by recognition and abortion of the malformed embryo.

Apart from the uncommon genetic grounds, the most reliable evidence of high risk of malformations is in respect of maternal rubella and administration of certain drugs during pregnancy. The risks following consumption of drugs such as thalidomide are not accurately established, but they are undoubtedly high and the remedy is obviously to avoid their use. A common infection such as rubella presents a more difficult problem. The probability of early death or serious malformation following infection in the mother during the first twelve weeks of pregnancy is at least one in five and may be much higher;[8] on present knowledge abortion offers the only means of avoiding the high risk of a malformed birth. But although rubella and thalidomide frequently lead to malformations, they are not common causes

[8] Rawls, W. E., Desmyter, J. and Melnick, J. L. *J. Am. Med. Assoc.*, 1968, **203**: 627–31.

of malformations, and if all abnormalities attributable to these and the few other recognized teratogenic agents were eliminated by prevention or abortion, the effect on the incidence of malformations in livebirths would be small.

It is for this reason that so much attention is focussed on methods of identifying malformed embryos or fetuses. The proportion which draw attention to themselves, for example by the presence of hydramnios, is small, and the observation is usually made late in pregnancy when all that is possible is early induction of labour. A number of conditions – spina bifida, hydrocephalus, achondroplasia, abnormalities of bone – can be seen on x-ray, but this approach would require routine radiology which would be undesirable. The difficulty which limits the methods of prenatal investigation so far available – chemical, chromosomal, radiological – is that to be fully effective they would need to be applied in all pregnancies, but if so applied the risks in some cases would outweigh the benefits. The answer appears to lie in two directions. One is through identification of mothers whose risk of having an abnormal birth is sufficiently high to justify the hazards of investigation. This requirement is considered to be met by women who have had a child with Down's syndrome, or are at an advanced age, although there are differences of opinion about the age above which amniocentesis should be carried out. The other approach is by investigations which do not require material from the uterus. It is illustrated by estimation of the level of alpha-fetoprotein in maternal serum as evidence of neural tube defects in the fetus, a screening procedure now used commonly in Britain. These methods are of great importance if we conclude, as I believe we must, that on present evidence the prospects for preventing malformations by avoidance of conception or elimination of teratogenic agents are not bright.

From birth At least in the immediate future, it seems likely that the problem of malformations will continue to present from birth at about its present level. The difficulties should not be exaggerated. Most malformations raise no large issues for society or medicine, either because they offer no threat to the quality or duration of life, or because they are incompatible with survival. The proportion of the malformed who present serious problems is certainly less than 1 in 6 and is probably less than 1 in 10.

There is no dispute concerning the treatment of most malformed children. No one is likely to question the desirability of closing a cleft palate, or of surgery in congenital heart disease where an operation offers the prospect of normal life to patients who would die early if untreated. The problem arises where the outcome of treatment is the survival of a child with a serious physical or mental handicap, and this occurs particularly in malformations of the central nervous system.

In such cases the desirability of treatment can be examined with two considerations in view: the quality of the life which is prolonged by medical intervention; and the price paid in care of the handicapped, particularly by close relatives, but also by the community at large through provision of social, educational and medical services.

It is at this point that controversy begins, and it is important to distinguish between those whose principles allow no account to be taken of quality of life or cost of care – they hold that life should be prolonged without regard for the consequences – and those whose conscience allows no escape from the dilemma presented by some of the most serious malformations. This distinction can readily be made by reference to anencephalus, which is characterized by gross maldevelopment of the brain and death before or within a few hours after birth. Logically, anyone who thinks that no account should be taken of the consequences, should agree that it would be a proper goal of medical research and practice to provide a vegetable existence for the anencephalic, without regard for the cost to public services or the unimaginable distress of close relatives, particularly the parents. But those who cannot accept this grotesque interpretation of humanism must face the formidable problem of deciding with what degree of handicap and at what price to the community they would consider it undesirable to intervene to prolong life.

In relation to these issues, spina bifida has come to have something of the status of a test case. This condition is the result of failure of the spinal cord to close during prenatal development, and by closing the lesion the surgeon is able to prolong the lives of certain children who without treatment would die soon after birth. Some of these children will be paralyzed and incontinent for the rest of their lives, in certain cases mentally retarded also. Moreover, most of those who will be paralyzed are known from birth to be irreversibly paralyzed.

Since the patient cannot represent himself, and a careful weighing of the complex medical, ethical and other issues is almost impossible for the parents, the decision in such cases is often influenced by the doctor. Unless he takes the uncompromising view that all lives must be saved without regard for the consequences, he has to decide whether to recommend intervention, having regard for the criteria referred to above – the effects of survival on relatives and the community and the quality of the life prolonged.

As judged by the number of places needed in special schools, the cost to the community of surgical intervention in all operable cases of spina bifida would be large. Decision is most difficult when something like a normal life can be achieved at high cost. In the case of spina bifida, however, what is achieved is not a normal life, but a cruelly handicapped one. A life indeed of such quality that many would think it wrong to prolong it even if no price were paid by the community in supportive services.

This raises what is perhaps the most difficult problem posed by the treatment of serious congenital deformities. On what basis can a judgement be made that the quality of life will be such that it should not be prolonged? The test which many people apply is this: Would I wish myself to live, or to have my own child survive from birth with such a handicap? When confronted by the prospect of lifelong paralysis from spina bifida, some of us have no doubt about our answer.

Mental Handicap

Since mental handicap may be caused not only by defective genes and uterine hazards, but also by numerous influences after birth, its aetiology is perhaps more complex than that of any other prenatal or postnatal abnormality. Nearly all the major determinants of disease may be involved: defective genes (of several types); early and late uterine hazards; birth injury; infection; economic, social and psychological influences; trauma; old age, and, for good measure, iatrogenesis. Indeed almost any severe disease or disability, directly or indirectly, may result in intellectual impairment.

When considering ways in which the problems of mental handicap can be dealt with, it is particularly important to keep in view the distinction between the physiological types which are at the lower end of the distribution of intelligence in the general population – mentally retarded, as it were, by definition – and the more severe and less common pathological types which are defective because they are ill. At the risk of slightly over-emphasizing the distinction, it might be said that one is essentially an educational and social problem, whereas the other is biological and medical. Largely because of deficiencies of services, the two have become administratively confused, for the physiological cases are often found in hospitals and the pathological ones are sometimes without medical and nursing care.

With such a serious defect, where the prospects of cure are small and the need for care is great, it would probably be agreed that primary prevention, through avoidance of conception, would be the ideal solution if it could be achieved by methods that were effective and ethically acceptable. The most severe cases of mental handicap are infertile. Attempts have been made to discourage or prevent reproduction of defectives, for example, by sterilization or segregation during reproductive ages. Some American States have laws that permit or require sterilization of people affected by a number of conditions which include idiocy, imbecility and feeble-mindedness. Apart from ethical objections to this approach, the results are not impressive, since the great majority of the mentally handicapped of all grades are born to parents who are not themselves affected, the reduction in the frequency of the defect by preventing all known cases from having children would not be large. In principle a few prospective parents whose children would be at risk from single-gene or chromosomal abnormalities could be identified, but this would require widespread screening of the general population which, with uncommon conditions, would be impractical on economic and other grounds. Moreover, when such people can be identified, most of them prefer to become pregnant and accept the possible need for abortion of an affected fetus rather than to remain infertile.

Secondary prevention, by abortion of abnormal embryos identified during pregnancy, is more feasible, and is being used in prevention of Down's syndrome, where the increased frequency of the abnormality at high maternal ages provides a basis for screening. However, many cases, probably the majority, occur in young mothers. In time, no doubt, it will become possible to identify several genetically determined forms of severe mental handicap, and screening methods will continue to improve. However, the problems of applying such procedures in rare conditions will remain. But the most serious restriction on both primary and secondary prevention arises because in the majority of cases of mental handicap there are no physical abnormalities to be detected. The physiological types are essentially an expression of man's genetic variability, and their recognition and removal during pregnancy is neither biologically possible nor ethically desirable.

Because of the limited scope for preventive procedures, the problems of mental handicap, like the overlapping problems of congenital malformations, are likely to continue to present from birth at about their present frequency. In a few examples, treatment is potentially curative, as in the case of dietary control of phenylketonuria and the use of thyroid extract in cases of cretinism. (Although in these diseases there are difficulties: the treatment of phenylketonuria requires lifelong care and supervision, and a child born a cretin may respond physically to thyroid therapy but is unlikely to reach the average level of intelligence.) In most pathological cases, however, cure of the serious and often multiple disabilities (for example in Down's syndrome) is almost inconceivable, and treatment is at best palliative. In the common physiological cases, as Penrose noted acidly, mental defect is 'merely the expression of normal variation in the intellectual capacities of members of the human species, and to speak of cure is absurd'.[9]

While it is obviously desirable that methods of prevention and treatment should continue to be explored, in the foreseeable future they can be expected to have limited success, and the frequency of mental handicap is unlikely to decrease. For although the incidence at birth is not rising – it may even be falling slightly – with the decline of infant and child mortality many people who formerly would have died in infancy now survive to adult life. It is particularly significant that an increasing number outlive the parents and relatives who have looked after them from birth, and they often need institutional care in later life.

Two major problems which arise in relation to the mentally handicapped are the medical and nursing care of those who are ill, and the education, training and employment of the much larger number who are free of physical disease. The approach to both problems is prejudiced by three difficulties: confusion between the roles of hospitals and community services; defects in the organization of hospital services; and the general failure of society to come to terms with the problems of the handicapped.

The trend of progressive opinion concerning the hospital's responsibility for the care of the mentally subnormal was well expressed in a Ministry of Health paper which stated: 'In the absence of complicating conditions, such as severe physical disability or disturbed behaviour, the severely subnormal patient who has been adequately investigated and treated ought not to be primarily the responsibility of the hospital services for long-term care. Ultimately, when facilities outside hospitals are fully developed, continued hospital care will be necessary only for patients who require special or continuous nursing and for those who, because of unstable behaviour, need the kind of supervision and control provided by a hospital'.[10]

It is well recognized that because of deficiencies of community services many patients are admitted and retained unnecessarily in hospitals. However, there are considerable differences of opinion about the proportion who could in practice be discharged. Some people appear to believe that with improved services most patients could be taken from hospitals into the community, whereas Penrose once remarked that anyone who thinks that the hospital population can be reduced rapidly is living in a fool's paradise. Here it is necessary to distinguish between what is desirable in principle and what is possible in practice. Some years ago an assessment

[9] Penrose, L. S. *The Biology of Mental Defect*. London, Sidgwick and Jackson, 1963: 268–95.

[10] Ministry of Health Memorandum. *Improving the Effectiveness of the Hospital Services for the Mentally Subnormal*. 1965, **104**.

was made of the feasibility of discharge of subnormal hospital patients drawn from the City of Birmingham. Approximately one third were thought not to need hospital care, but only about one fifth were considered suitable for discharge to their own homes or, more commonly, to hostels.[11] The difference between the estimates is accounted for by the fact that some patients judged not to need hospital care cannot in practice be discharged, particularly after prolonged periods of residence in an institution which has in fact become their home. However, it must be remembered that the present situation is the result of serious and long-standing deficiencies – inadequate assessment and treatment; admission of patients who should not be in hospital (usually because they have no home); retention of patients who should have been discharged; and lack of alternative facilities providing educational and occupational opportunities. It can hardly be doubted that with fully developed medical, educational and welfare services, the number of patients in hospital could be reduced below the Birmingham estimates. What is needed is to restrict the hospital responsibility to what is essentially the medical task, and to assign to educational and welfare authorities patients who need education, training, employment and a home.

A second difficulty arises because hospitals for the subnormal are separated, often widely, from other types of hospitals. This segregation has resulted largely from historical circumstances and has many disadvantages: the heterogeneity of patients, with inclusion of many who do not require hospital care; the difficulty of attracting staff, particularly professional staff (doctors, nurses, occupational therapists) to isolated institutions; excessive hospital size (partly a consequence of staffing difficulties); insufficient research in hospitals remote from major research centres; and long distances for relatives and other visitors to travel. These consequences of isolation point to the need to unite mental subnormality hospitals with other types. So long as the patients include large numbers who require no medical or nursing care, this proposal is unrealistic; but if responsibility were restricted to those who need hospital care, the way would be open to correct the historical accidents which isolated the mentally handicapped. In this way, and possibly only in this way, the standard of hospital care could be raised to an acceptable level.

The third difficulty to which I have referred is the failure of society to understand and come to terms with the problems of the handicapped. People with severe congenital disabilities, particularly those affecting the mind, are sometimes disliked, resented or even feared, as though their existence was in some ways a threat to the normal pattern of healthy life.

[11] McKeown, T. and Leck, I. 'Institutional care of the mentally subnormal.' *Brit. Med. J.* 1967, 3: 573-6.

These attitudes are reflected in low standards of care, and in attempts to get the handicapped out of sight and, so far as possible, out of mind, in isolated hospitals and special schools. It needs to be recognized that most severe cases of mental handicap result from the genetic lottery at fertilization, or are caused by the hazards of a prolonged period of intra-uterine life. 'High grade and borderline mental defect are phenomena which have come into prominence only since human life has become urbanized and industrialized. Civilized communities must learn to tolerate, to absorb and to employ the scholastically retarded and to pay more attention to their welfare. Subcultural variation, and the genes carried by the fertile scholastically retarded may be just as valuable to the human race, in the long run, as those carried by people of high intellectual capacity'.[12] For genes are not inherited with the same consistency as bank accounts, as Auden recognized when he wrote: ' "What a wonderful woman she is" Not so fast: wait till you see her son.'[13]

Low Birth Weight

If we exclude the malformed, whose disabilities result from their malformations rather than from their weights, infants of low birth weight are divisible broadly into two classes, according to whether the reduced weight is or is not preventable. The extreme reductions which are common in developing countries, and the smaller reductions seen in children of poor mothers in developed countries, are due usually to maternal malnutrition, often associated with ill health. Such problems can be relieved to some extent by dietary supplements before and during pregnancy, but their solution requires elimination of the poverty from which they arise.

An additional point has been made in chapter 4 about preventable low birth weight, namely, that if postnatal conditions are satisfactory, small or even moderate reductions are unlikely to prejudice the health and development of an otherwise normal child. This conclusion is based on the observations that in developed countries such differences are usualy eliminated after birth, and that in favourable circumstances twins perform as well as single births in intelligence tests at age eleven, in spite of their low birth weights. Perhaps the chief significance of moderate reductions of weight which are not attributable to causes such as multiple pregnancy and early onset of labour, is that they often arise in poor families in which postnatal conditions are likely to be unsatisfactory. It is important to remember that the newborn child is more vulnerable than the fetus. The problem must therefore be tackled, not only be raising birth weights, but by

12 Penrose, L. S. *The Biology of Mental Defect.*
13 Auden, W. H. *The Orators.* London, Faber & Faber, 1932: 40.

eliminating the poverty which leads to them and determines the unfavour-able conditions into which the children are born. The same considerations are even more important in relation to the severe deficiencies of weight in developing countries.

Low birth weights attributable to first pregnancy, multiple pregnancy and early onset of labour are obviously not preventable, and the chief requirement is to make adequate provision for the delivery and care of the children after birth. However this type of problem has been given a new dimension by recent advances in treatment of very low birth weight babies, some of whom may be physically or mentally handicapped.

In the case of the congenitally malformed, discussion was focused on the desirability of prolonging the lives of children who will *certainly* be handicapped. In the case of children of very low birth weight the ethical question is even more difficult: Is it right to prolong the lives of children who will *possibly* be handicapped. But we must put the size and nature of the problem into perspective.

In recent decades, and particularly in the last few years, there have been rapid advances in treatment of low birth weight infants. The improvement has been most conspicuous for children born after very short gestations (24–27 weeks) and at low weights. Forty years ago few were treated and not many survived; some were regarded as abortions. Even ten years ago mortality was high, 50 per cent for births under 1500 gms in the experience of several developed countries. Today, in the best units between 65 and 70 per cent survive without recognizable physical or mental handicaps, and while the possibility cannot be excluded that some will perform below the average, so far as can be judged within five or more years of birth (the extent of present experience) almost all of them are normal children.

To this point there are no large differences of opinion; it is generally agreed that the proportion of low birth weight infants who survive without handicaps has substantially increased. The question at issue is whether this improvement has been partially off set by an increase in the number of surviving handicapped children. Clearly, if more children survive and the handicap rate remains stable, the number with handicaps will rise. In Sweden, the incidence of cerebral palsy increased in the period 1971–76 when the more aggressive and specialized methods of neonatal care were introduced.[14] In the study based on data for several developed countries (referred to above), the handicap rate remained constant and relatively low (at 6–8 per cent) from 1956–60.[15] However, some physicians responsible

[14] Hagbery, B., Hagbery, G. and Olow, I. 'Germs and hazards of intensive neonatal care: an analysis from Swedish cerebral palsy epidemiology.' *Devel. Med. Child Neurol.*, 1982, **24**: 13–19.

[15] Stewart, A. L., Reynolds, E. O. R. and Lipscombe, A. P. 'Outcome for infants of very low birth weight: survey of world literature.' *Lancet*, 1981, **i**: 1038–41.

for premature baby units are convinced that the rate has fallen slightly in the last five years, and they believe that it will decline further. This improvement they attribute to better treatment and careful selection of patients who are to be treated.

Against this background the care of low birth weight infants may be said to raise two issues, one economic, the other ethical. The economic question is whether the high cost of facilities leading to survival of a considerable number of well children and a small number of handicapped ones is a wise use of medical resources. Stated in these terms the economic issue is essentially the same as the cost benefit assessment which arises in relation to all medical procedures.

The ethical issue is more difficult. Some people are concerned about methods of treatment which lead to the survival of seriously handicapped children, although many would probably regard this as a reasonable price to pay for the lives of a much larger number of well children. The problem which troubles others is a very different one. If the proportion of children surviving with handicaps is to be kept at a low level (say, 5–6 per cent), a much larger proportion (about 30 per cent of all babies under 1500 gms) must remain untreated. Many of these children would be severely handicapped if they lived, but the possibility cannot be excluded that, against the apparent odds, a few would be well. The methods in current use are therefore criticized by some on the grounds that they are too active and by others on the grounds that they are not active enough. And as already noted, the decisions are made more difficult by the fact that they are based on clinical judgements of the probable results of treatment rather than on certainties.

Recent experience with very low weight babies raises issues of the kind discussed in Britain by Kennedy in the Reith Lectures.[16] He criticized doctors on the grounds that many of their decisions are moral and ethical rather than technical. However, the examples he cited hardly bear this out, and it would be more accurate to say that many medical decisions are moral and ethical as well as technical. Whether to prolong the life of a low birth weight or handicapped child by medical intervention is certainly an ethical question, but the answer must be influenced by the resources and skill of the doctor and by an estimate of the possibility and extent of residual disability. However, most medical people would probably agree that 'the principle by reference to which doctors act must be the product of general discussion and debate.' The questions remain whether doctors wilfully usurp authority, and whether general principles can be established which would largely remove the need for medical decisions or advice when ethical issues are involved.

16 Kennedy, I. *The Unmasking of Medicine*. London, Allen and Unwin, 1981.

Doctors are neither better nor worse than other men, and in a situation in which power over others can be taken, undoubtedly some gladly take it. But I do not believe it is correct to say that most doctors have sought responsibility for the complex decisions with which they are faced, and I have no doubt that many would be relieved if some of the responsibilities could be removed from them.

The difficulty of establishing general principles which would eliminate or reduce the need for medical decisions is well illustrated by the care of malformed and very low birth weight babies. There is no dispute concerning the treatment of most infants who survive well or with trivial handicaps. The problem arises when the outcome of treatment is the survival of children with grave physical or mental defects. I believe that most doctors accept that such children should have simple care, although many would endorse the view expressed by Cardinal Griffin, that this does not mean that the lives of those cruelly handicapped must be prolonged by active medical intervention. Whether such measures should be applied they would regard as a decision chiefly for those affected, or, if they cannot represent themselves (as in the case of the newborn) for the parents. In practice the weighing of the complex ethical, medical and other issues is often impossible for the distraught parents, and they turn to the doctor for advice. But it is a distortion to say that doctors regard this as rightfully their decision, 'so that others intrude at their peril'.[17] Many doctors would be delighted if this burden could be removed from them, or if the profound issues could be resolved by public debate. But what can be written in general terms that will apply in all cases and remove the need for individual decisions? That all children who may have residual disabilities must be treated? Or that none should be? Or is there a definable position between these extremes which would not turn on medical judgements? The range of public opinion is as wide as the range of medical opinion, and when a severely handicapped child is born the anguished parents, assisted by their doctor, will still be left to make the critical decision.

Moreover some account must surely be taken of the doctor's religious and ethical convictions. A Catholic obstetrician cannot be required by public decree to perform an abortion which is against his principles, and a doctor who has himself suffered from a physical handicap can hardly be instructed to refrain from treating a malformed or low birth weight baby whose prospects he believes he can improve. What can be asked is that he has assessed accurately the consequences of his intervention before giving his advice: that in spina bifida, for example, he does not retire behind the euphemism 'acceptably dry' when evaluating the results of treatment of an

17 *Ibid.*

incontinent child whose mother has to live with the reality of persistent bed-wetting.

Conclusions

In this analysis of prenatal diseases, abnormalities determined at fertilization were considered separately from those determined during uterine life. This classification distinguished genetic diseases, for which the genes are a sufficient requirement, from diseases for which the genes are only a necessary requirement. The practical importance of this distinction is obvious: diseases determined at fertilization can be controlled only by replacement of defective genes, by avoidance of conception or birth, or by successful treatment; whereas abnormalities which arise later are potentially preventable by control of environmental influences. In our conclusions concerning disease control, however, it will be preferable to use a different grouping, taking together diseases which arise at and soon after fertilization, and separating them from conditions which appear in middle or later uterine life.

Diseases Determined At or Soon After Fertilization

At first sight it may appear inconsistent to group abnormalities which arise soon after fertilization with genetic diseases. Thalidomide and rubella are examples of teratogens which operate early in pregnancy, and variation in the frequency of some malformations – particularly anencephalus – by season, country and social class, is strongly suggestive of environmental influences. Moreover although progress in the discovery of teratogens has been slow, it is quite probable that a few more will be identified, although they are unlikely to be as frequent or as potent as thalidomide or rubella. But with due regard for this possibility, we cannot fail to be impressed by the fact that there is little evidence of reduction in the frequency of congenital abnormalities due to mental handicaps or malformations in the period when disease experience after birth has been transformed.

A solution to these problems is therefore unlikely to come from improvements in conditions of life; indeed some of them may increase, as a result of the use of pesticides, fungicides and the like. But many congenital abnormalities probably result from hazards associated with implantation and early embryonic developments and they may prove very difficult to identify and control. It is for this reason that abnormalities which arise soon after fertilization are grouped with the genetic diseases, on the assumption that they must be managed mainly by the same methods which depend on knowledge of their mechanisms – avoidance of conception, abortion or treatment.

Unfortunately the prospects for the methods of choice – avoidance of conception and successful treatment – are not bright. Few parents who transmit genetic diseases, malformations or mental handicap, are themselves affected. For some recessive disorders, tests for heterozygous carriers are not available, and when they are available they may be unrealiable or difficult to perform. Identification of carriers is possible in the case of a few common disorders, such as thalassaemia, and potential parents of affected children can be told about the risks of marriage and reproduction. But the general difficulty which besets this approach is that parents at increased risk – whether recognized by a genetic test or by the occurrence of a previous abnormal birth – often wish to become pregnant, particularly when an affected fetus can be identified and removed by abortion. For this reason, avoidance of conception is likely to make little contribution to the control of congenital abnormalities.

The same is true of treatment. There are a few conditions in which treatment can be said to be successful, particularly in some malformations of the heart. There are others in which its contribution must be acknowledged with reservations which are considerable (for example in cretinism and phenylketonuria) or very serious (as in spina bifida and thalassaemia). But for most disorders established at fertilization or early in embryonic life, successful treatment of the underlying disability is almost inconceivable, as in Down's syndrome, or is irrelevant, as in the common type of mental handicap where there is no physical abnormality to be treated. Successful replacement of defective genes, 'the ultimate achievement in genetic engineering', is unlikely to be possible within the period for which it is realistic to plan.

It is because of the restrictions on the other, and in principle, preferable approaches that attention is increasingly focused on antenatal diagnosis followed by abortion. Although some people have ethical reservations, this approach is generally accepted where the risk of abnormality is great, as in rubella infection, or where an affected fetus can be identified, as in Down's syndrome and thalassaemia. However, there are practical difficulties. In time the lack of reliable tests will no doubt be largely overcome, but the problem will remain of applying the tests in rare disorders whose discovery would require screening of all pregnancies. Moreover, the approach is not applicable to the most common type of mental handicap in which there is no evident physical abnormality.

It hardly needs to be said that the search for ways of preventing and treating serious congenital abnormalities should and will continue. This brief appraisal of their prospects suggests that antenatal diagnosis followed by abortion will have most to offer; but even with the use of this method, the frequency of most of the common disabilities at birth is unlikely to be substantially reduced. Attention, therefore, needs to be focussed increasingly on provision of care for the congenitally disabled: medical and nursing care if they are ill, and education, training and employment if they are mentally or physically handicapped. We also need to be concerned with the complex ethical issues which arise in relation to prevention, treatment and care.

Abnormalities Determined Later in Uterine Life

Most of the abnormalities which arise later in uterine life appear to be preventable, and the chief object of research and practice should be to identify and control the hazards to which the fetus may be exposed. Attention was drawn to them by the appalling mutilations from rubella and thalidomide, and several other potentially teratogenic agents are now known or suspected, among them radiation, alcohol, tobacco and drugs. These are influences which should be reduced or avoided at any time in life; but the fetus is particularly vulnerable, and advantage should be taken of this fact in health education, since a mother will often do for her child what she would not do for herself. Internationally, of course, the largest preventable prenatal problem is low birth weight, attributable essentially to maternal ill health and malnutrition.

The prenatal diseases determined later in uterine life require research and services which fall under the same headings as most diseases which arise after birth. Maternal ill health from malnutrition and related causes, is derived from poverty, and the measures needed for its elimination are well known if not always easy to apply. They are largely of an economic and political character. Abnormalities attributable to alcohol, tobacco, drug abuse and other health damaging behaviour are comparable to postnatal diseases of affluence, and the research need is of the applied type and largely behavioural. Reduction of infant and maternal mortality requires improved health care before, during and after labour. All of these problems have their analogues in postnatal life, but they are given particular poignancy before birth because of their impact on the child as well as the mother.

To summarize these conclusions: Some abnormalities which arise before birth can be prevented by control of the conditions which lead to them; but those established at or soon after fertilization cannot be managed in this way, and must be approached through knowledge of their mechanisms. In the foreseeable future, replacement of defective genes is unlikely to be successful, and with a few exceptions, neither prevention of conception nor curative treatment has much to offer. The approach which has been most successful is antenatal diagnosis, followed by abortion; but this measure is unlikely to reduce substantially the frequency of congenital abnormalities. The need for medical care and social services from birth will continue, and may increase because of the improved survival of the congenitally handicapped. Among the important problems to be considered is the ethical acceptability of some of the methods already in use: for example, reliance on abortion as an important weapon, particularly when a fetus is not certainly abnormal; treatment of very low birth weight babies, some of whom may be abnormal, or failure to treat them because of the risk of abnormality; the use of active measures to prolong lives which will be seriously handicapped.

8

Diseases of Poverty

'If we could know whence we have come and whither we are going, we would know better what to do and how to do it.'[1] In the health field there is no longer much doubt about whence we have come. The long debate of the eighteenth and nineteenth centuries concerning the origins and control of infectious diseases is at an end. We now know that the decline of the infections, and the vast improvement in health to which it led, resulted mainly from advances in conditions of life, supported in the twentieth century by immunization. In respect of one important aspect of whither we are going, there is not much room for dispute. Except for diseases specific to the tropics, the infectious diseases of developing countries can be largely prevented by well-known means. It must also be remembered that the diseases of poverty have not been eliminated from industrialized countries, where differences in health standards between rich and poor are almost as striking, and less excusable than in the Third World.

When we consider how much we know about the causes of disease, it seems surprising that improvement in health has not been more rapid, particularly in developing countries. There are large areas of the world where health today is no better than it was in developed countries before the eighteenth century; many children die within a few years of birth and most are dead before maturity. Moreover, on the basis of present policies the prospect of achieving everywhere by the year 2000 an acceptable minimum standard of health - say, infant mortality below 50 (per 1000 live births) and life expectation at birth above 60 years - cannot be said to be bright. In some countries the difficulties are compounded by extreme poverty, and by the prevalence of tropical diseases which were uncommon or absent from the developed world. Nevertheless, the rate of progress is also limited by failure to identify the main determinants of health, and to establish clear priorities in health activities.

[1] Lincoln, A. *The House Divided Speech.*

The failure to establish priorities is evident in health service policies. In general there is a much greater investment in the treatment of disease than in its prevention, but this has resulted from public demands and medical traditions rather than from assessment of the effectiveness, or even the humanity, of different approaches. The World Health Organization has made a commendable attempt to cover essential requirements by promoting the concept of 'primary health care'. But although this concept reflects admirably the spirit of the 'health for all' commitment accepted at the international conference in Alma-Ata in 1978, it is written in general terms which need to be developed in specific proposals. What should be the balance between preventive and therapeutic measures? Between, for example, the treatment of children with diarrhoea by rehydration therapy and reduction of their number by improvements in maternal and child nutrition? Because of the limits on resources it is unfortunately not a sufficient answer to say that both are necessary. Yet in health policies, the distinction between what is desirable and what is essential has still to be made.

An inspection of the research programmes of developing countries, as reflected in the work of their medical research councils, universities and health departments, will also show that there are no well recognized priorities. Indeed some research administrators go so far as to reject the idea of goal-directed research; they believe that the best results are achieved by finding able investigators and giving them their heads. As would be expected, the agenda which results from this approach, in its full or modified form, is unpredictable. Subjects for research could equally well be added or removed from the current lists, since there is no logical basis for their inclusion.

Another difficulty is that some of the most powerful influences on health are outside the influence of health administrations. Health services are normally taken to comprise the treatment and care of the sick, and the public health services which have developed since the nineteenth century. These included many services concerned with the prevention of disease and the promotion of health – environmental sanitation, communicable disease control, maternal and child health, school health, industrial hygiene and the like. But they do not include responsibilities related to the basic conditions of life – agriculture, housing, education, employment, economic policies – and health administrations have little or no direct influence on them. Particularly in developing countries, health standards are determined essentially by government policies as a whole, rather than by the limited range of services administered by health departments.

Let us consider now the services which need to be given priority if health is to advance rapidly. The decision is critical in the Third World, but it is also important for people in industrialized countries who are still exposed to the deficiencies and hazards which result from poverty.

The Third World

There are two sources to which we can turn for knowledge of the influences on health which require priority. One is the experience of developed countries during the last two centuries; the other is the experience of some developing countries which have made rapid progress in health in the last few decades.

The influences which have transformed health in industrialized countries were discussed in previous chapters and can be summarized here. This experience indicates that the improvement since the eighteenth century resulted mainly – until 1900 wholly – from the decline of mortality from infectious diseases. The *direct influences* which led to the decline of the infections were:

1 Increased resistance to infection, brought about by:

 a Improved nutrition, which was responsible for the advance in health in the eighteenth and nineteenth centuries when exposure to infection was increasing because of industrialization, expansion of cities and rapid population growth;

 b Immunization, which accelerated the decline of mortality in the twentieth century, particularly by reducing the pool of infectious people.

2 Reduced exposure to infection, through hygienic measures applied progressively from the late nineteenth century. The important developments were clean water, improved sewage disposal and, a little later, advances in the handling of food and improvements in housing. To a limited extent, exposure has also been reduced by treatment.

However, *indirect influences* were also important. As already noted, control of fertility came at the time needed to safeguard the advances from the effects of rising numbers. In England and Wales the population would have trebled by today if the birth rate had remained at its 1870 level.

But there were other important indirect influences, less clearly recognized. One was an increase in literacy: in England and Wales the introduction of compulsory education coincided with advances in water and sanitation and with the beginning of the decline of the birth rate. And more generally, it is an indication of increased public awareness that some of the most critical decisions related to health – increased productivity of the land, improvements in hygiene, limitation of numbers and advances in education – were all taken within a period of less than a hundred years. It is also evident that improved economic conditions underpinned the advances in nutrition and hygiene.

If there were no other knowledge to guide us, it would not be unreasonable to apply this experience of industrialized countries to the health problems of the Third World. In doing so, however, we would need to recognize certain differences. First, many of the countries are in tropical or sub-tropical areas where additional problems exist. Second, more is known now about the means of control of disease, and some measures – particularly immunization – are much more effective than they were at an early stage in industrialized countries. Third, for a number of reasons the time available for improvement in health is shorter, measured in decades rather than centuries according to the timetable accepted by the international community in Alma-Ata. And finally, the order of events is unlikely to be the same as in developed countries, where a century and a half of improved nutrition preceded hygienic and other advances, and the decline of the birth rate occurred at precisely the time needed to limit population growth.

Fortunately additional evidence is now available from a number of countries in the Third World which have made rapid advances in health: Sri Lanka, Costa Rica, India (Kerala State), China, Thailand, Cuba, Jamaica and a few others. Their experience has been examined in a number of books, papers and case studies, and the discussion which follows is based largely on this material. Use has also been made of data published in the annual reports of UNICEF and some other agencies. Inevitably the reports vary in scope and quality; some are concerned with a single country, others present comparative data; some deal with a single determinant of health, others with multiple influences.

For the purpose of assessing the main influences which contributed to the advances in health two reports have been particularly valuable. In 1984 WHO published case studies from five countries which described linkages between government departments and attempted to assess the relative importance of the influences which contribute to health.[2] In 1985 another conference sponsored by the Rockefeller Foundation also examined data from several countries and drew attention to the need for further research to clarify the relationships between different influences.[3] Unfortunately, this type of study is restricted by lack of data, particularly in longitudinal examinations over a period of time where the material for the early years is usually incomplete.

[2] World Health Organization. *Intersectoral Linkage and Health Development*. Geneva, Offset Publication No. **83**, 1984.

[3] Rockefeller Foundation. *Good Health at Low Cost*. 1985.

Infant mortality rates are the indices most generally available, but death rates are increasingly recorded for older children. There is less information about mortality in adult life, although age specific mortality rates are sometimes given in special studies. In many developing countries births and deaths are not reliably recorded, so that estimates of life expectation from birth are not available or must be interpreted cautiously. There is also a serious deficiency of both national and local data on morbidity.

A few general points are worth making at the outset. First, infant mortality rates are almost always higher in rural than in urban areas, and the urban rates differ relatively little between countries. Second, data for Sri Lanka suggest that as mortality declined, expectation of life increased more for women than for men: in 1921 life expectancy for men at birth exceeded that for women by 2.0 years; in 1972 the level for women was 2.8 years greater than for men. (However at ages 1 to 9 years, mortality was consistently higher for girls than for boys). Finally, evidence from Kerala State suggests that although mortality in infancy and childhood has fallen over several years, morbidity rates have changed very little.

On what may be regarded as the most basic observation and the starting point for further enquiry, the experience of the countries which have recently advanced is consistent with the conclusion based on industrialized countries: the improvement in health was almost entirely due to a reduction of deaths from infectious diseases. When examining reasons for their decline it will again be desirable to keep in mind the distinction between direct and indirect influences.

Nutrition Assessment of the nutritional status of populations, or even of individuals, is notoriously difficult. Where the total food supply is known – and usually it is not – because of variable losses in distribution, storage and use, it cannot be translated into a measure of average food intake. There are methods for measuring the food taken by an individual or a family, but they are time consuming and suitable only for research programmes. It is even more difficult to assess changes in nutritional status over a period of time.

In spite of these problems, the experience of the developing countries which have made rapid advances leaves no doubt that nutrition played a major part in determining mortality levels at all ages. However, the level of nutrition which is best for health is still not clear. Malnutrition affects the mental and physical development of children, and they become taller as countries become healthier and more prosperous. Nevertheless, in India there are differences of opinion on whether 'small' children should be regarded as diseased. But although there are many unanswered questions, a consistent conclusion from these studies is that nutrition was the single most important determinant of health.

Immunization   It is perhaps surprising that immunization appears to have contributed little to the recent advances in health. This is not of course because immunization is ineffective; but the reduction of mortality occurred in a period when vaccine coverage was still relatively low, and, as in industrialized countries, death rates had fallen because of other causes before vaccination became widely available. Indeed, as previously noted, the level of coverage in many developing countries is still very low.

Water supply and sanitation   were important influences in industrialized areas, but they do not seem to have been very significant in the countries that have recently advanced. The coverage of the population by supplies of clean water and safe sanitary measures was low in China, Sri Lanka and Kerala – lower indeed than in many other developing countries – although their death rates were well below average levels. There is some evidence that improved personal hygiene, especially in relation to food preparation and handling, can lead to substantial benefits. Water supplies are costly to install and frequently break down, so that simple measures such as hand washing and the use of soap may be valuable in the early stages of hygienic development.

Control of fertility   In spite of large differences in culture, religion and economic and social conditions, the countries that have advanced in health all achieved a considerable degree of control of fertility. The limitation of numbers and associated birth spacing undoubtedly contributed largely, if indirectly, to the reduction of mortality, particularly in infancy and childhood. There is some evidence that birth limitation may not always be essential in the first phase of improvement. In Costa Rica infant mortality fell for half a century when there was little change in the birth rate, but it declined even more rapidly when there was an abrupt reduction of the rate at the end of this period.

Education   This was an important influence in all the countries that made rapid progress in health. Here it is important to distinguish between general education and education related to health and disease: it is the level of general education that was closely linked to advances in health.

The extent of primary education can be expressed in various ways: the percentage of the sexes at different ages who are literate; the proportion of children registered in schools; the number of teachers per head of population; and the proportion of the population who have completed a stated number of years of education. The last is probably the most useful index and it is available for several countries.

Many countries show a close relation between health advances and the extent of primary education. Almost without exception the education of women was thought to be a more powerful influence than the education of men, although male education is also important, since it raises earning capacity.

The evidence suggests that primary education of children is more effective than that of adults. However, its impact may be delayed for many years, until the female children have become mothers, since infant mortality was more closely correlated with education rates twenty years previously than with current rates.

Although primary education is important to health, the results from secondary education appear to be even more impressive. Primary education is of course an essential basis for secondary instruction, and at an early stage of development there is no justification for developing secondary and higher education at the expense of primary instruction.

Economic development It goes almost without saying that economic development is an important indirect determinant of health. However this statement needs some qualification. Prosperity, as indicated by the gross national product or per capita income, is not always essential, since in some circumstances the distribution of wealth and the use of resources may be as significant as their creation. Among the countries that have advanced rapidly, China, Sri Lanka and Kerala State are poor as judged by per capita income, and some others are in the mid-range of income of developing countries. By contrast, there are countries with a high per capita income, of recent origin and generally based on oil, which have shown little improvement. A low level of economic activity does not prevent progress in health and economic wealth does not ensure it.

Provision of health care services It is well known that the treatment and care of the sick absorb most of the resources devoted to health services, and it is widely believed that this is justified by their contribution to health. In Costa Rica it was shown that a rapid fall in mortality rates followed the expansion of health care in 1970, and it was concluded that this development was more important than socioeconomic influences. However, at the time when better care was provided, the country was already well advanced economically and in provision of education and food, so that the population was at a level at which it could benefit from improved personal care. This suggests that the timing of personal services is important, and they have their greatest impact after some other developments have taken place.

Equity of access Equity of access to the determinants of health has been strongly emphasized by the World Health Organization in its approach to 'health for all'. It was regarded as an important feature in all the countries that have advanced, and was thought to apply to all the major influences. In Kerala and Sri Lanka, for example, the poorest sections of the community are no better off than the poor in some other countries, but they receive a larger share of the available wealth. There is also more general access to education. Although these countries are poor, even in relation to developing countries as a whole, the available resources and services are more evenly distributed and no section of the population is seriously deprived.

Political and social will   It is impressive that the political and social will to improve health existed in all the countries that have advanced. In some this originated from the people themselves, and is largely the result of prolonged education which led to awareness of basic human rights. In other countries, and notably in China and Cuba, the political will is centrally directed and organized on behalf of the people. However it was mobilized, this motivating force was vitally important for the equitable distribution of resources that was essential for progress.

Although these conclusions from developing countries that have recently advanced are incomplete, they are on the whole consistent with those drawn from experience of the developed world. They suggest that in a Third World country which seeks to progress rapidly, an essential requirement, and in a sense the starting point, is the political and social will to bring about improvement in health. The initiative may come from the government, as in China, or from the people, as in the State of Kerala, where they have become aware of the possibility of a better and healthier life. This awareness is largely determined by the general level of education, both primary and secondary, and particularly by the education of women. All the countries have achieved some degree of equity in access to the resources that determine health. Economic development is of course desirable, and in the long term essential for sustained improvement. Nevertheless, some poor countries have reached higher standards of health than others that are wealthier (or, more accurately, less poor), by their determination to advance and their acceptance of more even distribution of resources as the necessary means.

The experience of both developed and developing countries leaves no doubt about the over-riding importance of nutrition as the major determinant of health, and where resources do not permit an immediate attack on all the basic influences, it seems right to give priority to nutrition. Chapter 5 discussed international studies of the reasons for food deficiencies and malnutrition in different countries and regions; what is needed now is a close analysis of the problems within each country and of the solutions that are possible. This will require an assessment of the national food situation – sources, adequacy, distribution – and identification of malnourished people and the reasons for their deficiencies.

If standards of nutrition are to improve, it is clearly essential to reduce the rates of population growth in many Third World countries. It is sometimes said that limitation of numbers is unnecessary because food supplies can be expanded indefinitely, but this conclusion is inconsistent with experience in the developed world and in developing countries that have recently advanced. Without exception they have achieved some control of fertility. And the point, although theoretical, is worth making, that if only one change could be made in a country at an early stage of development, strict limitation of numbers would arguably have the greatest effect on health.

One of the most interesting observations on the handful of developing countries referred to above, is that their advances in health were achieved without substatial improvements in water supplies and sanitation, and before there was adequate coverage of the populations by vaccination. This indeed is a repetition of experience in industrialized countries where improved nutrition also preceded other measures. There is of course no doubt about the effectiveness of hygiene and vaccination, and a further advance in health can be expected when the services can be included. Unfortunately, as previously noted, the general provision of clean water and sanitation is beyond the means of many developing countries, but protection of children by immunization is usually within their reach.

It may seem surprising, even perverse, to leave to the end of this appraisal the service that people value most highly, the treatment and care of the sick. It is vitally important; yet it does little to reduce the frequency of disease or to improve the general standard of health in the community. There is no more difficult task related to health planning than achievement of a just balance between preventive and therapeutic measures, between assistance to those already in need and efforts to reduce their number. It is a problem that needs to be considered separately in each country, and perhaps the only general observation that should be risked is that in many countries too high a proportion of health resources is devoted to treatment services.

Tropical Diseases

As many developing countries are in tropical and sub-tropical areas, their diseases include both infectious and non-communicable diseases that were absent or uncommon in the developed world. Southwood has discussed reasons for their prevalence in tropical environments. 'Firstly, the abundance and variety of other primates, often living in proximity to man, provide a rich and diverse reservoir of hosts from which the parasites may transfer to man; thus there is the opportunity for many zoonoses. Secondly, there are the abundance and variety of insects and other disease vectors. Their variety is a reflection of the faunal richness of tropical environments; their abundance throughout the area arises in part from the climate. In the absence of a winter period, breeding may occur throughout the year and the generations are short and over-lapping.'[4] Primates suffer from a great range of diseases – helminthic, protozoal, microbial and viral – which may be transferred to man; but not all parasites of man are derived from primates or from the prehominoid past. 'Leishmaniasis is shared with rodents and carnivores, plague with rodents, and hydatid disease with dogs'. The Gambiense form of African trypanosomiasis, formerly thought to be exclusively a human infection, has been found in pigs.[5] The diseases are transferred to man (and, occasionally, from man to other animals) not only by vectors, but by the use of common facilities such as waterholes and rubbish bins.

In spite of the abundance and variety of parasites and vectors in the tropics, tropical diseases can be said to belong to the diseases of poverty because, like other infections, they are largely determined by conditions of human life. Their prevalence and geographical distribution are related to economic and social factors as well as to climate: to malnutrition, multiple infections, inadequate housing, ecological circumstances and human beliefs and practices. Exposure is greatly influenced by human behaviour: for example, large scale forest clearance in Latin America, notably in the Amazon basin, and in South East Asia, carries a high risk for leishmaniasis and malaria respectively; gem mining in Asia and gold mining in Brazil carry a risk for malaria, as does tin mining in Zaire for schistosomiasis.[6] If resources were available the risks could be greatly reduced: the diseases have almost disappeared from temperate zones (where admittedly the problems were less difficult); affluent travellers can safely visit tropical areas; and well-to-do tropical residents are effectively protected. Indeed in the extreme case, if sufficient wealth were available human populations could avoid areas where the risks of tropical diseases are great, just as they avoid polar or desert regions that are uncomfortable or unsafe.

But although tropical diseases have much in common with other infections, there are important differences in degree if not in kind. They do not

[4] Southwood, T. R. E. 'The natural environment and disease: an evolutionary perspective.' *British Medical Journal*, 1987, **294**: 1086–9.

[5] UNDP, World Bank, World Health Organization *Tropical Disease Research*, Geneva, World Health Organization, 1987.

[6] *Ibid.*

respond, or do not respond adequately, to the relatively simple improvements in conditions of life which transformed experience of infectious
diseases in developed countries, and greater emphasis is needed on other
measures – control of vectors, vaccines, drugs, diagnostic tests and
treatment – measures which depend on biomedical knowledge. Moreover,
the diseases, agents, vectors and reservoirs are constantly changing in
response not only to natural evolution but also to attempts to control them.
These characteristics have led the World Health Organization to create a
tropical disease research programme (TDR), with the aim of focussing a
broad range of scientific interests on the diverse problems presented by the
diseases themselves, the infectious agents that cause them, the vectors that
carry the agents and the animal reservoirs that harbour them. The diseases
selected for initial study comprise over 20 different entities in six groups:
malaria, schistosomiasis, the filarial diseases (including onchocerciasis), the
trypanosomiasis (both African sleeping sickness and the American form,
Chagas' disease), the leishmaniasis and leprosy.[7]

In this context a brief reference should also be made to the important
group of non-communicable diseases that are specific to the tropics, the
hereditary anaemias – sickle-cell anaemia and the thalassaemia syndromes.
They are genetic diseases determined at fertilization, and their control
requires assessment of the measures discussed in chapter 7 – replacement of
defective genes, avoidance of conception, elimination during pregnancy
and treatment. After considering these possibilities I concluded that in the
foreseeable future elimination of affected fetuses is the most promising
approach.

Industrial Countries

In chapter 5 we noted that there are still large differences in standards in
health between poor and well-to-do people in developed countries. These
differences are now present in some non-communicable diseases, but they
are most marked in the traditional diseases of poverty – malnutrition and
infectious diseases. There is little doubt that in developed countries the
greatest advance that could be made in health would be elimination of the
inequalities that still exist.

Is it more effective to attempt to eliminate poverty, or to tackle individu-
ally the multiple problems to which it gives rise? A good deal can be done
by attention to specific hazards and deficiencies, as in the case of the school
meals, food supplements and subsidies which contributed so much to
preservation of health in some countries during the Second World War. It

_____
[7] *Ibid.*

has been said that infectious diseases in the Third World can be prevented by immunization, and it is sometimes implied that it may be unnecessary to deal with the malnutrition or the underlying poverty. Quite apart from the questionable morality of this conclusion, it seems most unlikely that the multiple and complex influences which now cause disease can be removed without an attack on their common source, the gross inequalities in the distribution of resources. In the very different conditions of developed and developing countries, Scandinavia and Kerala have pointed the way.

Infectious Diseases in the Future

In discussions of the changing pattern of disease it is often assumed that the infections were the diseases of the past and that the non-communicable diseases which have partially displaced them are the problems of the indefinite future. Except in relation to conditions determined before birth these assumptions are questionable; it is unlikely that the infections were predominant before the historical period, and in time the roles may again be reversed. For if we are correct in thinking that the new pattern of non-communicable diseases is largely the result of environmental and behavioural changes associated with industrialization, many of the influences could be removed without prejudice, and in some cases with benefit, to the quality as well as to the duration of life. To assume that behaviour will not be modified for health purposes is not only to take a low view of human educability; it is also to overlook the enormous changes that have occurred in the last few centuries. After all, it is not long since our ancestors practised infanticide, burned witches, prescribed capital punishment for minor offences and employed young children for fourteen hours a day in mines and factories.

Man's long term relation to his parasites is a much more open question. Where it is possible to prevent contact with them, as in the case of organisms spread by water and food, there is no reason to doubt that control will continue to be effective. We cannot have the same confidence about diseases caused by organisms normally found in the body, or transferred from other animals by vectors such as the mosquito, tick or snail. J. B. S. Haldane said that the Almighty must have been inordinately fond of beetles. On the evidence of the ability of the common micro-organisms and disease vectors to resist the measures directed against them, He must have had a strong attachment to invertebrates in general. In Hiroshima, where human beings were devastated by the multiple effects of the atomic bomb, the earth-worms survived unharmed near the hypocentre, and after a prudent withdrawal for a few days the flies and mosquitoes returned in greater numbers.

Moreover the disappearance of an infectious disease provides no certainty that it has gone forever. Smallpox, for example, is said to have been eradicated; but as there are closely related viral infections of other animals – monkeypox, camelpox, goatpox and buffalopox – we can hardly believe that the virus, or others capable of evolving into it, has disappeared forever from the animal reservoirs from which presumably it initially emerged.

Predictions about future health trends over long periods are notoriously unreliable, but my own guess is that a hundred years from now it is more likely that wholemeal will have replaced refined flour, that environmental hazards will be strictly controlled, that the dairy industry will have contracted to a modest size, that smoking will be assigned a place somewhere between spitting and the taking of hard drugs – about as unpleasant as the one if not quite so lethal as the other – and that diseases such as influenza, malaria and the common cold will have been eradicated.

At this point it should be emphasized that the threat from infectious diseases is by no means restricted to the Third World. Their rapid decline since industrialization has led to some complacency, and it is widely assumed that serious infections will not reappear, or that if they do they can be controlled. On an evolutionary time scale the three centuries in which they have declined is a trivial period, and it would be foolish indeed to believe that man's relation to micro-organisms has been finally stabilized. Attention has recently been drawn to the risk of further pandemics from airborne infections, for example, from new strains of influenza – A virus arising as zoonoses.[8, 9] But the most dramatic evidence of the continued threat from infectious diseases is the appearance of AIDS, a disease caused by the human immunodeficiency virus (HIV), which within a few years has spread widely through the world and in some countries has already reached epidemic proportions. This experience is instructive as well as alarming, since it raises question concerning the source, conditions of spread and possible means of control of new or recurring serious infections.

AIDS is believed to have originated in Africa as a viral infection acquired from other animals which were probably simian. It is spread most commonly through sexual intercourse, but also by perinatal infection from mother to child, and by injection of infected blood, usually by drug abusers. It was first recognized in 1981, when it appeared to be limited to a

[8] Burnet, M. *Natural History of Infectious Diseases*, Cambridge, Cambridge University Press, 1962.

[9] Beveridge, W. I. B. *Influenza: The Last Great Plague*. London, Heinemann, 1977.

group characterized by minority sexual practices within a single nation. By October 1986, 33,217 AIDS cases were reported to WHO from 101 countries drawn from all continents. The largest number, 28,592 (86 per cent of the total), were from the Americas; Europe had 3,245, Africa 1,008, Oceania 317 (all from Australia and New Zealand), and Asia 55.[10]

Because of lack of diagnostic capacity and reluctance to notify the condition, the numbers reported represent only a small fraction of the AIDS cases. The true dimensions of the disease were more accurately assessed in the United States, which had 90 per cent of the cases reported from the Americas. The government estimated that between 1 and 1.5 million US residents were HIV infected, and that about 270,000 AIDS cases will have occurred by 1991. Using a transmission model, Knox has calculated that if an effective vaccine does not become available, on the basis of present sexual practices there will be 20,000 to 40,000 deaths per year in the United Kingdom.[11] But no area of the world is more heavily infected than Africa. Because of deficiencies of surveillance and diagnostic facilities, and the lack of a clear definition of AIDS, it is difficult to assess the size of the problem, but it is believed that Africa has the highest proportion of the population infected and the largest number of cases.

The pattern of spread of the disease is different in different parts of the World. In the United States, as in several other countries of the Americas, Europe and Oceania, the characteristic disease pattern is described as western: it is primarily an infection of homosexual and bisexual men and of intravenous drug abusers. In Africa, although the basic modes of transmission are the same (sexual, perinatal and blood contact), heterosexual spread (man to woman and woman to man) is common, and intravenous drug abuse is almost unknown. And because heterosexual transmission is usual, pregnant women are frequently infected and pass the virus directly to their children before, during or after birth. It is said that in some parts of Africa 10 per cent of pregnant women are HIV seropositive and 5 per cent of all new born children may be infected.

In Asia the position so far is quite different. The disease has only recently started to appear, and a few cases have been reported from India, China, Taiwan, Hong Kong, Japan and Thailand. They are believed to have arisen from imported blood and blood products, or from sexual transmission by male and female prostitutes. There is little evidence of HIV infection in the general population.

This brief history of AIDS illustrates several points previously mentioned

[10] Assard, F. and Mann, J. M. *AIDS - An International Perspective*. Geneva, World Health Organization Features, No. **103**, 1986.

[11] Knox, E. G. 'A transmission model for AIDS.' *Eur. J. Epidemiol.* **0392-2990**, 1986: 165-77.

in relation to the sources and spread of infectious diseases. First, although infective organisms do not cross readily from other animals to man, occasionally they do, and the outcome is determined by the character of the organism and the conditions it encounters. The usual result is the death of the parasite, so that the infection ends at this point. But it may cause acute illness, or survive for short or long periods without causing much disease or spreading widely unless it meets the conditions it requires. The malaria parasite and the tubercle bacillus, for example, are believed to have existed in prehistoric times; but malaria became a serious problem when large numbers of people were placed near to stagnant water in warm climates where the mosquito could breed, and tuberculosis became a common cause of sickness and death when the industrial towns provided ideal conditions for the spread of the bacillus – large, ill-fed populations residing and working in close proximity. We shall never know where or when the AIDS virus first infected man; but it is a disease spread readily by personal contact, and it is evident that conditions in the last quarter of the twentieth century – sexual promiscuity, drug abuse and frequent movements of people within and between countries – have met the requirements for its transmission. And although good nutrition is not an adequate defence against the infection, it may not be without significance that the disease is most common in the continent where malnutrition is widespread.

Against the background of experience of infectious diseases it is possible to suggest the general lines of the defences that can be erected against them. They fall broadly under three headings: reduction of exposure; increase of resistance; and treatment.

Reduction of Exposure

An obvious requirement is to prevent or reduce contact with infective organisms so far as possible, and the feasibility of this approach depends largely on the ways in which they are spread. It is relatively easy (in developed countries) to prevent exposure to water-borne diseases; it is more difficult to control those spread by food, animal vectors and personal (including sexual) contact; and it is usually impossible, particularly with large, aggregated populations, to prevent transmission of airborne infections. Moreover, as Dubos noted, 'the microbial diseases most common in our communities today arise from the activities of micro-organisms that are ubiquitous in the environment, persist in the body without causing any obvious harm under ordinary circumstances, and exert pathological effects only when the infected person is under conditions of physiological stress.'[12] In general, the success of reduced exposure has

12 Dubos, R. *Man Adapting*. New Haven, Yale University Press, 1971: 164.

been greatest by application of hygienic measures which have prevented transmission of organisms spread by the faecal-oral route, but control of vectors is also important, particularly in tropical diseases, as is modification of personal behaviour in relation to a disease such as AIDS.

Increase of Resistance

Increased resistance was the main reason for the reduction of infectious deaths in the last two centuries, and it is still the most potent defence in the Third World today. Improvement in nutrition has been the major influence; but an important contribution is increasingly being made by immunization and may also come in future from the control of stress.

The contribution that immunization can make was examined in a WHO report which assessed the impact of biomedical research on health care.

Infectious diseases, whether of bacterial, parasitic or viral origin, can be considered in a world-wide perspective to be the most important group of diseases to attack. In the present state of knowledge this effort is likely to be more successful than those directed at many other diseases. The major factors behind this supposition are the advances in molecular biology and immunology. The knowledge about the chemistry of micro-organisms and the mechanisms of their replication offer possibilities to produce vaccines specific for important structures responsible for infectivity of the micro-organisms. At the same time, this way of attacking the problems of vaccine production decreases or eliminates unwanted side-effects of vaccines. Recombinant-DNA technology has provided a means of preparing immunogenic material at reasonable cost. A particular advantage with this technology is that deletion mutants which lack certain virulent genes can be prepared. These mutants will be antigenic, but safer than vaccines prepared by procedures currently used. Another possibility for vaccine production involves utilization of subunits or components of micro-organisms. Such vaccines will contain parts that are antigenic but lack components that may cause infections or other unwanted side-effects. Still another approach is preparation of vaccines containing crucial, antigenic peptides. The possibilities of this procedure are difficult to assess at present; there is a problem of protein conformation, that these peptides must resemble in a three-dimensional way the structure of the whole protein in the membrane of the micro-organisms.

Vaccines may also be constructed as anti-antibodies which act as antigens and elicit immune response. There is already experience from experimental systems that anti-idiotypic vaccines are effective in viral diseases such as hepatitis, influenza and polio and in parasitic diseases such as trypanosomiasis.

When parasites are considered, for example, malaria, it can be assumed that vaccines will contain proteins from different stages of the evolution of the parasite. By such a design it will be possible to attack the parasite at different stages of its life cycle.

A problem with vaccines that is not yet satisfactorily solved is that of adjuvant. To make the vaccines optimally effective adjuvants are needed. It can be assumed that the research on the regulation of the immune system will provide knowledge about suitable and effective compounds that stimulate the immune system.

In discussing vaccine production the role of the use of monoclonal antibodies should not be overlooked. Monoclonal antibodies constitute an invaluable instrument to define antigens relevant for induction of protective immunity or mediation of pathologic response. They can be employed in purification of antigens to be used as vaccines.

Overall, the prospects of controlling infectious diseases in the coming decade seem good and can be attributed mostly to breakthroughs in biomedical research such as recombinant-DNA and monoclonal antibody techniques. It should be added that basic biomedical research also will provide better instruments for vector control. Suffice it to mention elucidation of the chemical structures of many sex attractants in insects.[13]

Immunization of the world's children is increasing quite rapidly: in 1987, 50 per cent were protected against tuberculosis, diphtheria, whooping cough, tetanus, poliomyelitis and measles; ten years earlier the proportion was 5 per cent. Unfortunately the level of vaccine coverage is lowest in developing countries for measles and neonatal tetanus, the two diseases which cause most deaths. WHO emphasizes that it is essential to immunize children even if they suffer from minor illnesses or are malnourished. But although the presence of malnutrition does not make it undesirable to provide immunization, it is equally true that the availability of immunization does not make it less necessary to prevent malnutrition.

It has been suggested that stress plays an important part in the origin and course of many diseases, including the infections, and that for the immediate future the most valuable weapon the public possesses is the knowledge that in so far as stress is a cause, precipitant or risk factor in disease, it is not such because of the impact of the stressor, but because of the reaction of the individual to the stressor.[14] It is not easy to distinguish between the impact of the stressor and the reaction to it; but overlooking this difficulty, it is suggested that those identified as at risk can learn to avoid stress or, better, to react less violently when exposed to it. Techniques such as relaxation, meditation and biofeedback are available for this purpose.

One can recognize the importance of stress without accepting the generality of these conclusions. Multiple influences are involved in the causation of diseases, and their relative importance is not the same in every

---

13 World Health Organization. *Health Research Strategy*. Geneva, 1986.
14 Inglis, B. *The Diseases of Civilisation*. London, Hodder, 1982.

case. For example, the rapid decline of tuberculosis in industrialized countries is more credibly explained by improvement in nutrition, reduction of exposure and treatment than by reduction of stress. In the Third World today, the provision of sufficient food, clean water and immunization would contribute more than other measures to the control of infectious diseases. Dietary changes offer the most promising approach to some intestinal disorders and possibly to the control of hypertension. The observation of a relationship between personality and proneness to lung cancer would not change the conclusion that elimination of smoking is the most effective means of preventing the disease. (If the concept of genetic proneness had been known in the nineteenth century, some people no doubt would have said that the best approach to prevention of typhoid would be to identify those who could safely drink polluted water). Indeed, in the light of experience of screening policies I am doubtful whether the division of a population into groups with greater or lesser risks of disease is very useful, except in the case of occupational and similar hazards. Selye, the pioneer of work on stress, clearly recognized the importance of controlling the origins of diseases as well as the response when he wrote: 'No disease is purely a disease of adaptation, any more than a disease of the heart or an infectious disease is a "pure disease" in which adaptive phenomena play no part. The term "disease of adaptation" should be used only when the adaptation factor appears to be more important than any existing pathogen itself.' This criterion is not met in lung cancer, constipation, obesity, tuberculosis and food poisoning, to give only a few examples.

Treatment

The treatment of a non-communicable disease could not be expected to reduce its frequency, but the treatment of a chronic communicable disease can limit the number of people who spread infection. This possibility is illustrated by treatment of venereal diseases, such as syphilis and gonorrhoea, and of an airborne infection such as tuberculosis.

The effect of treatment on the frequency of infectious diseases has been small, except in the case of tuberculosis. It was estimated that in England and Wales, chemotherapy lowered the number of deaths from the disease in the period 1948–71 by about half,[15] and since the infectivity of patients is quickly reduced by treatment, there was a substantial fall in the number of infectious people in the community. However it must be remembered that

[15] McKeown, T. *The Role of Medicine: Dream, Mirage or Nemesis?* Oxford, Basil Blackwell, 1984.

mortality from tuberculosis has declined from the early nineteenth century, and the greatest influence on its frequency was improved nutrition.

In summary: When deciding health policies, Third World countries can profit from the experience of a handful of developing countries which have recently advanced rapidly in health. This experience shows the need for acceptance by governments and people of the goal of improved health, and of the means required for that end – a more equitable distribution of resources and improvements in education, particularly of women. As in industrialized countries, the better health resulted from a decline of mortality from infectious diseases, brought about largely by improvement in nutrition. All the countries achieved a considerable reduction of the rate of population growth, an essential basis for the other advances. Coverage of the populations by hygienic measures (clean water and sanitation) and by immunization was low, and further improvement in health can be expected when these services are provided. The tropical diseases are also related to conditions of life determined by poverty, but raise additional problems which require greater emphasis on measures such as the control of vectors, vaccines, diagnostic tests, treatment and – in the case of the hereditary anaemias – the management of genetic diseases.

In industrialized countries, elimination of the inequalities that still exist is the greatest advance that could be made in health. These inequalities are the result of poverty, and their removal would be medically simple if politically difficult. A good deal can be done by attention to specific hazards and deficiencies (especially of food), but in view of the multiple effects of poverty on conditions of life as well as on health services, it is still questionable whether 'the masses will be healthy unless, to their very base, they be at least moderately prosperous.'[16]

Although the behaviour of parasites is almost infinitely variable, the threat from infectious diseases is determined largely by the conditions of human life. Experience of the last half century shows that most serious risks can be avoided by reduction of exposure or increase of resistance, but there are new and persistent infections that arise from ways with which change would be difficult or unacceptable: dense populations, foreign travel, contact with strangers, medical procedures and, remarkably, improved conditions which postpone infections until late life.[17] New or recurrent infections will continue to appear by transfer from other populations or from other animals, and control will depend on effective vaccination and treatment unless the conditions which enable the organisms to spread can be modified.

[16] Simon, J. *English Sanitary Institutions*. London, John Murray, 1897.

[17] Velimirovic, B. *Infectious Diseases in Europe*. Copenhagen, World Health Organization, Regional Office for Europe: 1984.

9

Diseases of Affluence

The analysis of disease origins in Part II led to the conclusion that most diseases are not inevitable; except when determined at or soon after fertilization they result from unhealthy ways of life and can be prevented if those ways be changed.

For almost the whole of his existence man was unable to manage his environment or limit his reproduction, and the chief causes of sickness and death were deficiencies of basic resources or hazards arising from the search or competition for them. These are still the main influences on health in the Third World, and in the poor of developed countries. In the advanced countries, however, it has been possible to exercise a considerable degree of control of the environment, and for the first time the benefits were not lost because of rising numbers. These advances led to the decline of infectious diseases; but, ironically, they have been associated with a new pattern of non-communicable diseases attributable to profound changes in the environment and in behaviour. The future level and pattern of health will depend largely on the extent to which these changes can be reversed or limited, in industrialized countries where they are already well established, and in the developing world where they are beginning to appear.

In the Preface to *The Doctor's Dilemma* Shaw summarized in a few words the requirements of prenatal and postnatal life: 'One should take care to get well born and well brought up.' In relation to health, in a developed country getting well born means starting life free of congenital disabilities, and getting well brought up implies exposure to a healthy environment and acquisition of personal habits consistent with the requirements of health. A perceptive fetus with these aims in view would be well advised to consult standardized mortality ratios, statistics which give the relative risks of death according to age, sex, marital status, occupation, location of residence and the like. It would come about as near to immortality as human genes permit by electing to become the wife of a rural clergyman; well-to-do but living frugally; fertile but with few children; physically active, but avoiding field sports, especially hunting; taking no drugs, alcohol or tobacco; and keeping to a diet low in salt, eggs, fat and sugar, and so rich in fruit, vegetables and grains that the addition of bran would be an indulgence.

Of course, we cannot all be wives of rural clergymen; nevertheless, it is possible to progress towards ways of life that retain the advances on which our present health largely depends, while removing some of the hazards that threaten health because they depart radically from the conditions for which our hunter-gatherer genes have equipped us. What is required is elimination of the effects of poverty without incurring the risks that have been introduced by industrialization and affluence.

When considering these risks it is useful to make a distinction between environmental and behavioural hazards. Environmental hazards are those that arise from the natural or man-made environment, over which an individual has little, and sometimes no direct control – working conditions, atmospheric pollution, road traffic. Behavioural hazards are determined primarily by personal actions – for example, smoking, drug abuse and overeating. The distinction is by no means always clear-cut; many environmental hazards such as road traffic are influenced by individual behaviour, and behavioural hazards such as diet, smoking and alcohol, are determined substantially by public policies. Nevertheless it is useful to distinguish the hazards that can be reduced or eliminated by governments and other public bodies, from those in which public policy can be implemented only by changing personal behaviour. For the individual the distinction is between risks that he can control by his own decisions and those that he can influence only indirectly by the use of his vote.

Behavioural Influences

Food

I think there is little doubt that food has been and remains the single most important determinant of health, particularly when considered in all its aspects: too much food or too little, the wrong food, and food infected by micro-organisms or contaminated by poisonous chemicals. The problems of food deficiency and infection arise as a result of poverty, so we are concerned here with the influences related to affluence: food excess, imbalance and chemical contamination.

Although large numbers of people are still undernourished, for the first time in history there are countries where the opportunity to overeat is no longer confined to a small minority. Weight standards based on insurance mortality statistics suggest that in England and Wales middle aged men are now on the average about 20lb overweight; American men are even heavier. Life insurance records provide impressive evidence of the effects of obesity: men who are more than 25 per cent above the average for their age and height have a death rate twice as high as those within 5 per cent. The differences are due to deaths from various causes, particularly ischaemic heart disease, diabetes, cerebrovascular disease, chronic nephritis and accidents. There is evidence that the problem begins in infancy; the overweight infant tends to become the overweight schoolchild and, later, the obese adult.

The question of food balance is perhaps the most controversial in the field of nutrition and the opinions of experts are often divided. Some years ago at a meeting in Oxford I sat at luncheon between two specialists, one of whom carefully removed all the cream from his pudding, while the other indulged liberally in a second helping. They were at least practicing what they preached, for the first taught that fat was the hazard and one should not take cream or eat an egg unless the hen had been exercised, whereas the second was the chief spokesman for the view that fat is no risk to health so long as one restricts the sugar. I know a distinguished physician who finds it impossible to believe that anything he likes could be harmful, and as he enjoys all food he sees no reason to limit consumption; he takes saccharin, not instead of sugar but in addition in order to sweeten it. One can see the point of the remark by a patient, that ideally every patient should have a doctor who suffers from the same disability. It must be difficult to treat, and still more to sympathize with someone who complains of dyspepsia if one has never had indigestion.

Although all differences of opinion about an optimum diet have by no means been removed, there is general agreement in the reports published in recent years by the World Health Organization and government and other agencies in the United States, Britain and other countries. Essentially they recommend reduced consumption of dairy products, refined sugar, meat, and (less insistently) salt, and increased consumption of fruit, vegetables, cereal grains, fish and poultry. Broadly the aim is to limit the amount of fat, particularly saturated fat, salt and sugar, and to increase fibre, carbohydrates and animal protein from sources other than meat. It should be noted that such a diet is very close to the one that would be recommended if we took as a guide the food available to our Pleistocene ancestors: they had no dairy products, salt or refined sugar; their calories were obtained from fruit and unrefined vegetables (mainly) and from meat derived from wild animals living in their natural habitats.

Lastly, we must consider the risks of chemical contamination. In recent years there has been an unprecedented increase in the quantity and variety of chemicals used in the production, preparation, preservation and presentation of food, and during these processes chemicals may get into food by accident or may be introduced deliberately.

Until recently, accidental chemical contamination on a large scale was uncommon, but today the risks are widespread. Harmful chemicals may find their way into foodstuffs during production, for many are used in agriculture to protect plants against animal, insect and fungal pests. More than a hundred preparations have been identified that are a serious hazard to agricultural workers. The antibiotics and hormones employed in animal husbandry also present dangers; for example, penicillin in milk of cows treated for mastitis may cause unpleasant reactions in sensitized persons and may lead to sensitization in others. Harmful chemicals may be introduced accidentally into food during processing and storage. Disinfectants, catalysts and bleaching and clarifying agents are all widely used in the food industry, and the possible contamination of canned foods by metals, particularly zinc and lead, is a matter for concern. Further difficulties arise from the pollution of fishing waters with industrial effluents containing mercury and other poisons. The disposal of wastes from nuclear processes is only the latest, if the most alarming, of the risks from contamination.

Fraudulent adulteration of food is no longer common, but chemicals have been added legitimately since the eighteenth century. Chemical manipulation to preserve and 'improve' food is now widespread and difficult to control. Recognized and permitted practices include the addition of antioxidants, moisture retaining agents and surface protections to preserve food; sweeteners, acidifiers and spices to heighten flavour; dyes, bleaching agents, clarifiers and glazes to improve appearance; and emulsifiers, thickeners and tenderisers to enhance consistency. It has been estimated that in a year each of us unknowingly consumes about three pounds of chemicals which are not natural constituents of food.

Smoking

There is probably no other hazard whose ill effects on health have been, or perhaps could be, charted as meticulously as those of tobacco. There are several reasons why it has received so much attention. First, it has been under investigation for almost exactly the period – the last four decades – in which the origins of non-communicable diseases have been seriously considered; until the end of the Second World War interest in the relation of behaviour and environment to disease was almost confined to the infections. Second, the large increase in the frequency of smoking has occurred in the present century, when evidence from national statistics and other sources was much better than that available for diet and reproduction, in which some of the major changes occurred in the nineteenth century. And third, the effects of smoking on health are so large and so obvious that they are accepted even by people who dismiss other features of behaviour as scarcely worth attention.

Nor can very much be changed by the trendy fashions in changed 'life styles', all the magazine articles to the contrary; dieting, jogging and thinking different thoughts may make us feel better while we are in good health, but they will not change the incidence or outcome of most of our real calamities. Everyone should stop smoking; but we are still obliged, like it or not, to rely on science for any hope of solving such biological puzzles as Alzheimer's disease, schizophrenia, cancer, coronary thrombosis, stroke, multiple sclerosis, diabetes, rheumatoid arthritis, cirrhosis, chronic nephilitis, and now, topping the list, AIDS.[1]

According to this interpretation the science needed does not include investigation of the relation between health and the basic conditions of life, and tobacco can only be regarded historically as a bizarre, and - in view of present smoking trends - temporary exception.

Those who have challenged the evidence on tobacco have done so mainly on three grounds, and since they are a decreasing number their views are of interest chiefly because of their bearing on the approach to other behavioural influences. First, it is said that the statistical association does not prove that smoking causes cancer. This objection is largely met by the strength of the association, by the observation that mortality from lung cancer declines in people who give up smoking, and - for those who find work of experimental animals more convincing than controlled observations in man - by the production of lung cancer in animals which have inhaled cigarette smoke.

A second objection is that smoking produces effects that are apparently non-specific, since it is associated with increased mortality from several diseases. However, there is nothing surprising in the observation that smoking, like other agents as different as alcohol, the spirochaete and psychological stress, should have multiple effects. Moreover cigarette smoke is not a single chemical agent.

Thirdly, it has been suggested that certain people are genetically predisposed both to smoke and to develop lung cancer, and thus patients owe their disease to their genes rather than to their smoking. This hypothesis was thought to be supported by certain physical and psychological differences between smokers and non-smokers; however it is inconsistent with the large increase in death rates from lung cancer during

---

[1] Thomas, L. Review of: *Becoming a Doctor: A Journey of Initiation in Medical School* by Melvin Konner. *New York Review of Books*, 1987, Number **14**: 6–11.

this century and with the rapid fall in mortality from the disease in people who have stopped smoking cigarettes.

Most people who have reviewed the evidence, taking account of the inconsistencies and doubts that have been expressed, have no hesitation in accepting the conclusion reached in a report of the Royal College of Physicians of London: 'The quantitative association between cigarette smoking and the development of lung cancer is most simply explained by a causal basis and no other explanation accounts for the facts.'[2]

The ill effects of smoking have now been shown in many other diseases, and the evidence was summarized by Doll on the basis of his own extensive experience: 'The avoidance of smoking alone would reduce the mortality from all cancers by about a third (including avoidance of not only the large majority of cancers of the mouth, throat and lung, but also a substantial proportion of the deaths attributed to cancers of the bladder, kidney and pancreas). It would almost eliminate chronic obstructive lung disease and the complications of peripheral vascular disease, would reduce the age specific mortality from acute aneurysm by at least three-quarters, and would probably lead to a small reduction in perinatal mortality in the poorer socio-economic groups.'[3]

The measures needed for the prevention of smoking were summarized in a report of the Royal College of Physicians of London: more intensive education, particularly of children; phasing out of tobacco promotion; restriction of smoking in public places; and increased taxation, particularly on high tar cigarettes.[4]

Reproduction

The overall effects of the changes in the pattern of reproduction during the last hundred years have clearly been good. By maintaining a balance between resources and numbers, the reduction of the number of births contributed powerfully to a higher standard of living and, indirectly, to improvement in health. The reduction of the number of unwanted births is the main reason for the rarity of infanticide which was once so common, and for the decline in the frequency of illegal abortion and the unpleasant complications to which it frequently gave rise. Fewer births and longer intervals between births have contributed to the health of mothers and children; and there have been some advantages in the delay of reproduction

[2] Royal College of Physicians of London. *Smoking and Health Now*. Pitman Medical, London, 1971.

[3] Doll, R. *Prospects For Prevention*. Royal College of Physicians, London, 1982.

[4] Royal College of Physicians of London. *Smoking and Health*. Pitman Medical, London, 1977.

to later ages, particularly in avoidance of pregnancies of very young and often unmarried women.

But there have also been disadvantages in the changed pattern of reproduction. At later maternal ages infant mortality is increased, and although the risk of congenital malformations is sometimes overstated, Down's syndrome is much more common at late ages. It has not so far been possible to establish a clear relation between the changes in reproduction and the major diseases of the reproductive system, except of course in the case of venereal infections, which must now be taken to include AIDS.

To look ahead, perhaps further than one can see, it is possible that the diseases related to reproduction provide examples of measures that society is likely to accept and to reject in the control of diseases determined by personal behaviour. If it were shown convincingly that breast cancer could be prevented by a return to early and more frequent pregnancies, it is unlikely that the change would be accepted; the benefits would be bought at too high a price, both in other effects on health and in their general influence on the established pattern of life. No such price would be paid for a change in sexual practices, and particularly if effective vaccination or treatment of AIDS is not in sight, many people would consider that the use of condoms, discrimination in the choice of sexual partners and care in the use of needles are a price well worth paying for prevention of the disease.

Physical Exercise

An investigation of sickness and mortality records of London Transport drivers and conductors in 1953 showed an inverse relation between physical activity and coronary artery disease: drivers had more coronary disease than conductors; their disease appeared at an earlier age and was more frequently fatal. The conclusion that this result was due to variation in physical activity was confirmed by similar findings in a comparison of the experience of government clerks and postmen, and by an examination of mortality in a wide range of occupations in national statistics. Later investigations have confirmed the conclusions, and have provided an explanation by showing that physical inactivity leads to raised levels of blood pressure, blood lipids and insulin activity. It has also been shown that the risks can be reduced by frequent and vigorous walking.[5]

That people will change their personal habits to protect their health is perhaps more evident in physical exercise than in any other influence. All types of activity, from walking to marathon running, have become more

[5] Leon, A. S., Conrad, J., Hunninghake, D. D. and Serfass, R. 'Effects of a vigorous walking programme on body composition, and carbohydrate and lipid metabolism of obese young men.' *Amer. J. Clin. Nutrition.* 1979, **32**: 1776-87.

popular, and in the United States, always in the forefront of advance, there are places where one is at as much risk from joggers and cyclists as from motor cars. Perhaps the chief question that arises in relation to health is the type of activity that is advisable at different ages. If we take as our guide the customs of our nomadic ancestors, it seems certain that if well they were physically active throughout their lives, but it is unlikely that they voluntarily faced extreme demands, such as those imposed by competitive squash, bicycle tours and marathon running. The type of exertion for which our cardiovascular system was presumably genetically selected is walking, the life long activity of hunter-gatherers and peasant agriculturalists, on the flat or on hills according to the nature of their terrain.

Alcohol

Although alcohol is a major health and social problem, as there is no adequate measure of its effects on mortality and morbidity it is difficult to assess its size. An indirect indication is proved by death rates from cirrhosis of the liver: the rate is ten times higher in France, where average consumption is a pint a week in adults over the age of 15, than in the United Kingdom, where the amount is about a tablespoon a day, to a Frenchman hardly more than a medicinal dose. But mortality from cirrhosis is only a small part of the effect on death rates: suicides are much more common in alcoholics than in others, and about a quarter of the drivers killed in road accidents have blood alcohol levels above the statutory limit.

It is even more difficult to assess the amount of ill health due to alcohol, either from its direct effects on heavy drinkers or its indirect effects on others. The kinds of morbidity caused by alcoholism include chronic gastritis, cirrhosis of the liver, polyneuritis and mental illness (depression, changed sexual habits, delirium tremens, and Kursakow's syndrome). The World Health Organisation defined alcoholics as 'those excessive drinkers whose dependence on alcohol has attained such a degree that they show a noticeable mental disturbance or an interference with their mental and bodily health, their interpersonal relations and their smooth social and economic functioning; or who show prodomal signs of such developments'. According to this broad definition there are about 150,000 alcoholics in Britain of whom about a quarter (3 per 1000 of the adult population) show physical and mental deterioration.

The ways of preventing alcoholism have been discussed extensively and they include most of the approaches that have been advocated for the control of smoking: increased taxation; restriction of sale and advertisements; severe penalties for drinking and driving. But there is an important difference between smoking and drinking which has a considerable bearing on the long-term problems they present. If a hundred people start to smoke, most will become addicts and they will pay a heavy price in health loss; if a hundred people start to drink only a minority will become alcoholics, and the proportion who do is susceptible to reduction by the influence of social customs. The balance between costs and benefits is therefore quite different in the two cases, and while our successors may judge that the world would be better without tobacco, they are unlikely to forgo the pleasures and some health benefits from alcohol used judiciously. If this assessment is correct the long-term goals will be to eliminate tobacco and to prevent the misuse of alcohol.

Environmental Hazards

In their contribution to health in the past, the environmental measures introduced progressively from the second half of the nineteenth century were second only to improvements in nutrition. However, many well-recognized hazards associated with housing, atmosphere, traffic, insect vectors and working conditions are far from being eliminated, while others inherent in contemporary life have not been fully assessed or, in some cases, recognized. In developing countries effective control of the environment has scarcely begun. The discussion which follows will be limited to developed countries and will be concerned with only two aspects of the environment – the home and the place of work.

The Home

The association between ill-health and adverse living conditions is more immediately obvious than the relation between contaminated food or water and disease, but it is also more complex. People who live in unsatisfactory houses are usually poor, and it is difficult to separate the effects of bad housing from other adverse influences associated with poverty. Broadly, however, there are three main ways in which housing may affect health: through the structure of the house; through overcrowding; and through the location of the house in relation to other influences and amenities.

Badly built, dilapidated and poorly equipped houses are the direct cause of much ill health. Without an indoor hot water supply the spread of infection is facilitated by accumulation of dirt and refuse and the presence of vermin. When cooking facilities are inadequate and the larder is an unventilated cupboard under the starts, there is likely to be wasteful buying, an ill balanced diet and increased risk of food-borne infection. Uneven floors, steep stairs without handrails, bad lighting and dilapidated furniture and household fittings, lead to accidents in the home, particularly in young children and old people.

When large families live together in one room during the daytime and sleep several to a bedroom, opportunities for the spread of air-borne infection are greatly increased. Overcrowding may also have harmful psychological effects. When people are living too close together, instability and frustration due to clashes of temperaments and interests are inevitable and lack of privacy makes it impossible to hide these conflicts from children. Overcrowding in bedrooms – children with parents, older with younger children and brothers with sisters – may lead to emotionally disturbing sexual experience. The schoolchild has nowhere to play or study and the adolescent is not encouraged to bring friends into the home. The wheel comes full circle when young couples cannot afford a house of their own and are forced to spend the formative years of their married lives in the overcrowded houses in which they were born.

The ill-effects of substandard houses are often augmented by the lack of social and recreational amenities in the neighbourhood, and by the many adverse influences that arise from poverty and unemployment. Children play on the streets and in derelict houses, and adolescents meet at street corners and in public houses. These problems arise not only in pockets of bad housing in the older parts of industrial towns, but also in some housing estates built between the two World Wars with little regard for the need for amenities.

Although the association between poor living conditions and ill health seems self evident, there is little numerical evidence of the precise part played by various features of bad housing in the causation of sickness, disability and death. There are two reasons for this: bad housing has multiple effects on physical and mental health, and it is very difficult to separate its effects from those due to other consequences of poverty. Nevertheless, improvements in home conditions have undoubtedly contributed significantly in the twentieth century, and further improvement is needed if health is to continue to advance.

In large cities the rehousing of people from slum clearance areas presents many problems. The choice lies between blocks of flats in clearance areas – attractive to architects and planners but not to many of the people who have to live in them, new estates near the edge of cities which extend the urban sprawl, and satellite towns which provide a long term policy with its own difficulties. Whatever the site, the need is not only for new houses, but also for a new community with a life of its own. The provision of shopping and community centres, schools and health centres, playing fields, open spaces, public houses and churches, should be as much a part of a rehousing scheme as provision of bathrooms, bedroom space and facilities for preparing, cooking and storing food. A balanced community should take account of the needs of the young and the old, of small and large families, and it should make provision for growth and change.

The crux of the problem is to provide accommodation that an unemployed person or low wage earner can afford. The cost of satisfactory housing, like the cost of education and medical care, puts it beyond the reach of large sections of the population. It is therefore essential to lower housing costs, and to provide assistance through various forms of state subsidy. The opportunity to lower costs has come in some countries through the release of land formerly required for agriculture, and with good architecture and careful planning it should be possible to provide a solution which meets aesthetic as well as social and health needs.

The Work Place

The control of hazards in the working environment has two main aspects. The first is the need to protect people against dangerous substances, and since the respiratory tract is the common portal of entry to the body from industrial poisons, this requires above all control of atmospheric pollution. The second aspect is less precise but not less important; it is to protect workers from accidents, and to control the physical environment, particularly the heat, light and noise. The basis on which these objectives should be approached were outlined by the first medical inspector of factories in England and Wales. 'Until the employer has done everything – and everything means a good deal – the workman can do next to nothing to protect himself, although he is naturally willing enough to do his share. . . . If you can bring an influence to bear external to the workman (that is, one over which he can exercise no control), you will be successful – if you cannot or do not, you will never be wholly successful.'

These statements imply that responsibility for control lies essentially with the employer, and that protective devices that depend for their use upon the 'will or whim of the worker to use them' (respirators, goggles, washing facilities) can never be completely effective. Five principles have been recognized for control of occupational health hazards:

1 Substitution. The most fundamental approach is to change harmful materials and methods for safe ones. But although substitution is the ideal means of eliminating or controlling a hazard, it is often the most difficult to put into practice. There may be no suitable substitute, and an alternative when available may require extensive alterations in an industrial process.
2 Isolation. If a dangerous process cannot be changed for a safer one, the obvious precaution is to isolate it so that few or no workers

come into contact with it. This important principle is widely used throughout industry.

3 Ventilation. Good ventilation is essential to the health, and sometimes to the life of people working close to industrial processes that produce or use harmful dusts, mists, fumes or gases; it also adds greatly to the physiological and psychological comfort of indoor workers, whatever their occupations. When production of a dangerous substance is very localized, control by ventilation may be adequate, but when atmospheric pollutants are produced over a wide area (as in foundries, steel works and coal mines), the problem of their removal is technically much more difficult and may require the design and installation of extensive and expensive extraction plant.

4 Personal protection. In a few unusually dangerous occupations none of these methods of control can be applied, and the only satisfactory alternative is to provide this worker with personal safety appliances. In effect this is an application of the isolation principle, enclosing the worker rather than the toxic process. Except in such uncommon circumstances, protective clothing and appliances should not be the first line of defence against an unhealthy working environment.

5 Supervision. The four principles outlined above depend for their effective application upon supervision of the health of workers in relation to the environment in which they work. Codes of safe practice are required, and government inspection is necessary to ensure that employers comply with health and safety regulations.

Since the eighteenth century some enlightened employers have carried their efforts to provide safe, healthy and even attractive working conditions far beyond statutory requirements. But in general it is true to say that health supervision at work is one of the least satisfactory features of health services in developed countries.

Non-Communicable Diseases in the Future

In chapter 8, I questioned the conclusion that the infections were the diseases of the past, and that the non-communicable diseases which have partially displaced them are the problems of the indefinite future. I gave reasons for believing that some infectious diseases will persist, and I must now consider grounds for thinking that non-communicable diseases are likely to decline. They clearly will not do so as a result of treatment, so that the forecast rests on the belief that many of the behavioural and environmental influences that lead to the diseases will in time be brought under control.

An important step in this direction will come from general recognition that most non-communicable diseases have resulted from changes in conditions of life that have occurred in the last two centuries. Until recently many common causes of sickness and death were regarded as genetic diseases, and research was focussed almost exclusively on disease mechanisms. The last few decades have seen a beginning of interest in disease origins, stimulated by the impressive evidence of the effects of smoking. A change in the concept of non-communicable disease origins will lead to enlargement of interest in the relation between environment, behaviour and disease. We naturally search for the influences that we believe are there to be discovered.

If preservation of health requires changes, some of them major, in ways of life, two questions are certain to arise: What evidence is needed before public action is justified? And would considerable changes in the environment and behaviour be acceptable?

Evidence Required For Public Action

It is sometimes suggested that action cannot be taken to modify influences which may promote or damage health until evidence of their effects is complete. For this reason some would say that it would be unacceptable to change national food policies, to prohibit certain kinds of television advertising, to control suspected hazards in industry, to restrict the use of potentially dangerous drugs or to attempt to modify behaviour, except in the case of cigarette smoking where the grounds are considered to be sufficient.

It is fortunate that this requirement was not always imposed in the past. When Snow protected a London population from cholera in the mid-nineteenth century by removing the handle of the Broad Street pump, the evidence of the relation between the disease and the water supply was anything but complete; indeed neither micro-organisms nor tests of significance had been discovered. If thalidomide had not been withdrawn on the basis of an observed association between the drug and limb deformities and when knowledge of teratogenesis was very deficient (as it still is), many thousands of children would have been born with malformations. If the argument that an association does not prove causation and only experimental evidence is conclusive had been accepted, quite a number of people who found the relation between cigarette smoking and lung cancer sufficiently convincing would have died of the disease before beagles had been taught to smoke. And during the last World War, if the limited foods then available had not been distributed judiciously by rationing, subsidies and supplements, the health of the population would have been much less satisfactory than in fact it was. Yet it was not then, nor is it now, possible to specify with any precision the nature and mode of operation of the nutritional influences which were important.

Other examples could be cited in support of the view that action is often needed to protect and promote health in circumstances where the evidence is less than complete. Moreover, in many cases it is questionable whether within the foreseeable future it can be made complete. To assess precisely the respective roles of diet, exercise and smoking in the causation of coronary artery disease, a massive human experiment would be needed, with division of the population into multiple experimental and control groups. Such an investigation would take a long time and would present formidable ethical, technical and administrative difficulties.

In the light of such difficulties I believe it will often be desirable to act on the basis of high, or even moderate, probabilities, on what has been called 'a burden of prudence' rather than 'a burden of proof'. When applying this principle, however, we should distinguish between the levels of evidence needed for private and for public actions. Parents can act to protect their own or their children's health on evidence which would not be considered sufficient to justify public action. For example, they might think it right to encourage their children not to smoke, to avoid white bread and to limit their consumption of foods and drinks containing sugar, at a time when none of these practices is publicly prohibited. The level of proof needed for public action is a different question and has no single answer. Nevertheless, it should be recognized that conclusive evidence of harm or benefit is often an unrealistic requirement.

Acceptability of Changes in Ways of Life

In general, it is easier to control environmental hazards than those that arise from personal behaviour, and in the last century considerable improvements have been made by stricter supervision of working and living conditions. This progress will continue, as new risks are recognized and as public opinion becomes increasingly intolerant on aesthetic as well as health grounds of the pollution of the atmosphere, the addition of industrial and domestic wastes to seas and rivers, and the use of poisonous chemicals in the production and manufacture of food. In some cases the hazards will bring their own solutions: for example, it is hard to believe that cars will continue to be sold to as many people as can afford to buy them when traffic has reached a standstill, as it almost has in Tokyo and some other cities. With the expected rates of population growth traffic problems will be even more acute in some of the enormous cities of developing countries, and it will be less difficult to limit the numbers of cars than the numbers of people.

The problems presented by environmental hazards are epitomized by the use of nuclear energy for the provision of power and the production of weapons, the most bizarre examples of the application of man's intelligence to the dual problems of existence and co-existence. Who would have guessed that his best idea for preventing war would be to make its effects so widespread and so frightful that if it occurred no one would be safe? Or that the aggressive postures of two antagonists would be unaffected by the certain knowledge that if they fight both will lose? But perhaps the most serious threat is not from the accumulation of nuclear weapons in the hands of a few large powers, where conceivably they can be controlled, but from their possession by an increasing number of smaller nations which will make their own decisions about when to use them. If these weapons had been available to some of the countries that have been at each other's throats in recent decades, can there be much doubt that they would have been used?

The widespread development of nuclear power illustrates the conflict of opinions and interests which often beset environmental hazards. Since scientists who understand the technology are widely divided in their judgements about the balance of benefits and risks of nuclear power, it is obvious that the evidence is inconclusive. But if nuclear power is not developed on the advice of those who believe it is unsafe, if they are wrong there will be an economic loss; if it is used on the advice of others who believe it is safe, if they are mistaken there may be another nuclear accident like Chernobyl. This is an extreme example of issues which arise from environmental developments, when the evidence is incomplete, as it often is; there is a choice between convenience and financial interests on the one side and risks of sickness and death on the other.

Many people who can accept the need for public intervention in control of the environment, are deeply suspicious of attempts to modify personal behaviour. It is often said that this would be an unreasonable intrusion on the rights of the individual, and that any such attempt would be certain to fail. These objections are well illustrated by smoking, on which opinions are perhaps stronger than on any other habit.

It is said that an individual must be free to decide whether he wishes to smoke. But he is not free; with a drug of addiction the option is open only at the beginning, so that the critical decision to smoke is usually taken, not by consenting adults but by children below the age of consent. The main question confronting society is not whether smoking by adults should be prohibited; it is whether it is acceptable to induce children to become addicts at an age when they neither know nor much care about the associated risks.

The same logic should be applied to other aspects of personal behaviour which are known to be important to health. It is not suggested that we should be required to exercise, to limit consumption of alcohol, sugar and dairy products, to change from white to wholemeal bread, and to avoid most self-prescribed drugs and some of the physician-prescribed variety, beneficial as all these measures would undoubtedly be for our health. But it is not inconsistent with respect for personal freedom to attempt to create an environment which encourages people to do what is good for them and to avoid what is bad. It seems particularly reprehensible to do the reverse, as in seeking ways to induce people to damage their health by smoking for no other purpose than to sustain revenues and profits.

The conclusion that personal habits cannot be modified arises from the application of too short a time scale. Before 1800 there was no convincing evidence that human beings would restrict their reproduction on a significant scale, yet by the end of the century birth rates were falling throughout the western world. This change began among well informed people, but extended gradually to all sections of the population. With this evidence of modification of one of the most intimate features of behaviour there is no reason to doubt that in time other practices which are critical to health will also change. Indeed that they have begun to do so is evident in changes in diet, reduction of smoking and concern about food additives among well informed people.

However, much thought needs to be given to the means by which changes in behaviour can be brought about. The usual approach through advertisements, posters and public exhortations takes little account of the subtle influences which are shaping behaviour. Newspapers and television have no hesitation in exhibiting some of the most admired figures of our time with cigarettes in their hands or mouths, and television programmes in which bourbon is poured liberally at regular intervals to enable the principal characters the better to enjoy life or the better to endure it, have probably done more for the sale of alcohol than all the professional advertising. With unsolicited support of this kind it would not be surprising if tobacco and alcohol manufacturers regarded their vigorous defence of paid advertisements as no more than a minor skirmish designed to distract attention from the main event.

10

Conclusions

In the introduction to this book I compared the health scene to a complex jig-saw puzzle of which enough pieces are at last visible to enable them to be fitted into a recognizable whole. As the pieces have been scattered over several chapters, I will try now to bring them together. I shall look first at the complete picture, before summarizing the evidence on which the components are based.

The most fundamental conclusion is that except when determined at or soon after fertilization disease is not an inescapable attribute of the human condition; it results from unhealthy ways of life and can be prevented if those ways can be changed. The deleterious influences are of two kinds: deficiencies of basic resources, of which food is by far the most important; and exposure to hazards, which may be either natural, mainly from parasites, or man-made, from conditions that man has created for himself. Although the behaviour of parasites is almost infinitely variable, most serious risks from natural hazards can be avoided, because they are determined essentially by the conditions of human life; and man-made hazards are also potentially preventable, because they arise from the creation of a hostile environment and exposure to ways of life for which human genes are ill-equipped. Health depends primarily on removal of the long-standing deficiencies and hazards which led to the predominance of infectious diseases, without incurring the risks from non-communicable diseases that have appeared in the last few centuries as a result of the maladaptation and hazards associated with industrialization.

Disease History

The background of these conclusions is an interpretation of the determinants of health in the three main periods of human existence. In the period of hunting and gathering man was unable effectively to control his environment or limit his reproduction, but as he was well adapted to the conditions of life through natural selection, non-communicable diseases were rare, as they are in other primates living in their natural habitats. The shortness of life of hunter-gatherers was due mainly to food deficiency, acting directly through starvation and malnutrition, or indirectly through environmental hazards and response to infectious diseases.

Under agriculture there was a beginning of control of the environment, and an increase in food supplies led to a decline of mortality and expansion of numbers. But reproduction was not effectively restricted, and populations increased to the size at which food supplies became again marginal. As many of the basic conditions of life were unchanged, non-communicable diseases were still rare; but living together in large numbers and unhygienic conditions, human beings had inadvertently created precisely the conditions required for the propagation and transmission of many infective organisms. Infectious diseases became the predominant causes of sickness and death.

Industrialization extended control of the environment, and a large increase in food supplies and (later) reduction of hygienic risks together led to the decline of the infections. This time, however, the advance in health was not reversed by rising numbers, as it had been after the first Agriculture Revolution, because the nutritional and hygienic improvements were accompanied by a sharp reduction of fertility. Populations expanded, but at a rate more or less consistent with health requirements. However, industrialization created conditions of life far removed from those under which man evolved, and non-communicable diseases displaced the infections as the common causes of sickness and death.

In relation to the determinants of health, experience in the three major divisions of human life can be summarized by saying that in the first there was effective control of neither the environment nor reproduction; in the second, there was some control of the environment but not of reproduction; in the third there was further control of the environment and – for the first time – of reproduction, but insufficient control of conditions of life created by industrialization.

Disease Origins

In the light of this historical analysis, disease origins were examined by dividing diseases into three classes – prenatal diseases, postnatal diseases due to deficiencies and hazards, and postnatal diseases due to maladaptation and hazards. Prenatal diseases were considered separately because most of their causes are different and more intractable than those that operate after birth. But their separation has the disadvantages that some causes before and after birth (for example, smoking and malnutrition) are the same, and that certain diseases determined before birth are manifested postnatally, often late in life. For an understanding of disease origins designed to suggest means of control, a more fundamental distinction can be made between disorders determined at or soon after fertilization on the one hand, and all other disorders, whether determined before or after birth, on the other hand.

The diseases determined at fertilization are referred to here as genetic diseases, and it is confusing when they are taken to include the so-called common diseases, such as coronary artery disease and rheumatoid arthritis, for which the genes are a necessary rather than a sufficient requirement. Diseases established at fertilization are distinguished from others by the fact that they cannot be prevented by environmental (including behavioural) changes, but must be managed by avoidance of conception, elimination during pregnancy, treatment or replacement of defective genes.

For practical rather than theoretical reasons it seems prudent to regard as in the same class certain abnormalities (such as most congenital malformations) determined after fertilization but early in pregnancy. They arise at the time of implantation or early embryonic development, and while it is possible that some may be due to external influences such as infection or drugs, it seems probable that many have internal causes which will be difficult to identify and control. They are therefore unlikely to be prevented by environmental measures, and must be managed in the same ways as genetic diseases.

All other diseases have environmental as well as genetic components in their aetiology and are therefore potentially preventable. That this is not merely a theoretical possibility is evident from the facts that changes in health in the past were determined essentially by conditions of life, and that the modern transformation of health was brought about largely by environmental measures. To assess the possibilities of disease control we need to consider the nature of the major influences. They can be divided broadly into two classes, associated with poverty in the one case and – not quite so consistently – with affluence in the other.

For nearly the whole of human existence, as in the Third World today, numbers were excessive in relation to the resources available, and ill health was due mainly to the multiple effects of poverty. These effects have varied in different periods, but the constant and major determinant has been lack of food. There could be no more convincing evidence for this conclusion than the fact that in developing countries such as China and India (in the state of Kerala), which in a few decades have attained western standards of health, the advances are attributable almost entirely to improved nutrition; there were no substantial improvements in water, sanitation and personal health services, and immunization coverage was low. But the effects of poverty are also manifested through various hazards, particularly exposure to infectious diseases through defective hygiene and aggregation of large populations. The deficiencies and hazards derived from poverty are the major causes of sickness and death in the Third World today, and they are also largely responsible for the ill health of many poor people in developed countries. Moreover the difficulties will increase because of rapid population growth – the world's population is expected to double before it stabilizes – and the movements of people from rural to urban areas. It is painful to imagine what health conditions are likely to be on the streets of Calcutta or the outskirts of Mexico City in the twenty-first century, when the population of each city will be well above 20 million.

Chapter 6 presented several reasons for regarding the non-communicable diseases which have largely displaced the infections in developed countries as new diseases attributable to conditions of life brought about by industrialization: their incidence has varied in genetically stable populations; a racial group which has changed its location exhibits the disease pattern of the population with which it shares its environment rather than that of the population with which it shares its genes; the frequency with which children of the same family are affected is not much greater if they are genetically identical than if they are not; and – perhaps the most persuasive evidence – the diseases are uncommon or absent in hunter-gatherers and peasant agriculturalists, but begin to appear when they change from their traditional ways of life to the western life style. That the new disease pattern in the developed world is due largely to maladaptation is strongly suggested by the fact that profound changes in ways of life have occurred in the last few centuries when the genetic constitution of the human population has remained the same; indeed it has changed very little in the last 100,000 years, well before the appearance of Cro-Magnon man. However, some of the diseases cannot be attributed to maladaptation, for they are due to hazards created by industrialization – for example, road traffic, pesticides, atmospheric pollution – in which the risks are determined almost entirely by the new environment.

The long-standing deficiencies and hazards which led to the infectious diseases were the result of poverty; can the recent maladaptations and hazards responsible for non-communicable diseases be said to be due to affluence? Broadly, in developed countries the distinction seems valid; the eighteenth century was a watershed which divided the deficiencies of the past from the relative affluence of the industrial period. The opportunity for large numbers of people to over-eat, under-exercise and change their pattern of reproduction was created by a surplus of resources above essential requirements. But some of the hazards caused by industrialization – pesticides, food additives, industrial diseases – result from methods of producing wealth rather than consuming it, and are only indirectly related to affluence. Moreover the use of this term seems anomalous when some of the so-called 'diseases of affluence', such as coronary heart disease, diabetes and cancer of the lung, are becoming more common in poor than in well-to-do people. Nevertheless I have retained the term because it seems preferable to the usual alternatives (diseases of civilization; Western diseases) and contrasts with 'diseases of poverty' which describes accurately the conditions that prevailed everywhere until the last few centuries.

Disease Control

The advantages of separating diseases determined at fertilization or soon after from all others become evident when we turn from disease origins to consideration of disease control. These abnormalities cannot be prevented by environmental measures, and must be approached through knowledge of their mechanisms. I conclude that in the foreseeable future replacement of defective genes is unlikely to be successful, and that neither avoidance of conception nor curative treatment will have much to offer, desirable as these approaches undoubtedly are. The most effective procedure is likely to be antenatal diagnosis followed by abortion, and it has already been used successfully in populations in which an abnormality (such as thalassaemia) is common. Nevertheless this approach is unlikely to reduce substantially the frequency of congenital abnormalities such as the malformations and mental handicap, and the need for medical care and social services for the congenitally disabled is likely to continue at about the present level.

The prospects are much brighter for diseases determined later, usually after birth. Experience of some Third World countries that have recently advanced in health indicates that the diseases of poverty – chiefly the infections – can be prevented largely by improvement in nutrition, and experience of developed countries shows that additional advances can be achieved when exposure to infection is reduced by hygienic measures (clean water, clean food and sanitation) and when resistance to infection is increased by immunization. In developing countries the most urgent requirement for health is to improve nutrition, and to achieve this goal it will usually be necessary to distribute resources more equitably to enable people to buy food; to advance education, particularly of women; and to limit numbers. These were the measures that were successful in countries such as China and Sri Lanka. In developed countries the greatest advance that could be made in health would be elimination of the substantial inequalities that still exist between poor and well-to-do people. This is as much an economic as a medical problem, for removal of health inequalities requires redistribution of wealth, and probably depends finally on

inequality of Distribution of wealth

elimination of poverty. In the world today ill-health is due less to lack of resources than to their uneven distribution between and within nations.

NO yet Prevention of Life Disease

Experience with the non-communicable diseases that have arisen in the period of industrialization does not take us so far; indeed they might be said to be at the stage of the infections in the late nineteenth century, when their environmental origins were evident but the measures needed to prevent them had not been generally clarified and applied. We are still far from having achieved control of the hostile environment bequeathed by industrialization, or modification of the kinds of behaviour that lead to disease. Nevertheless public measures related to pollution, food additives, pesticides, road traffic, working conditions and the like are becoming increasingly strict, and it seems likely that at some future time, not too far distant, environmental hazards leading to non-communicable diseases will be as effectively controlled as those leading to the infections. We cannot have quite the same confidence about behavioural influences, whose modification may interfere with personal preferences. However, nearly everyone now accepts the need for effective control of dangerous drugs, most people would like to see smoking eliminated and alcohol consumption reduced, and many are prepared to modify their diet, physical exercise and sexual practices if they believe the changes are important for their health. The kinds of behaviour with which change would almost certainly be unacceptable are those related to essential features of modern life, such as small families, urban living, dense populations and foreign travel.

Very relevant

Some readers may find it remarkable that a book concerned with the origins and control of disease should have so little to say about its treatment. I have interpreted control as the solution of disease problems, and this can be achieved only by prevention or successful treatment. Unfortunately treatment of non-communicable diseases does not reduce their frequency, and treatment of the infections has contributed relatively little to their decline. Moreover even with successful treatment there is a formidable price to pay, in human suffering as well as in the cost of health and social services. The solution of disease problems is therefore concerned predominantly with prevention and in the future as in the past this is likely to come mainly from control of the conditions that lead to them.

End paragraph

But of course prevention does nothing for those who are already ill, the task with which western-style clinical medicine is chiefly concerned. Even if preventive measures were as comprehensive as we would like them to be, and so successful that we rarely encountered disease or disability due to a hazardous environment or to the twin threats of poverty and affluence, there would remain formidable problems determined before birth or associated with the end of life. Moreover, it would be a serious misrepresentation to suggest that all diseases due to deficiencies, maladaptation and hazards can be rapidly eliminated. Their prevention may be delayed, in some cases indefinitely, for several reasons: because the harmful influences are unknown (as in many neurological disorders); because they are multiple, and hence difficult to dissociate (as in coronary artery disease); because they are costly to eliminate (as are some occupational hazards); because their control requires changes in behaviour which people are reluctant to accept (as in cancer of the lung and cirrhosis of the liver); because they are biologically or technically complex (as are malaria, schistosomiasis and the common cold). For as long as the causal influences are not removed there will be need for treatment of diseases that are potentially preventable.

The knowledge on which such treatment is based must come mainly from biomedical research. Indeed nothing in the analysis of disease origins suggests that we can dispense with empirical investigations. There is no intuitive or metaphysical faculty that will lead to the solution of problems such as mental handicap, Alzheimer's disease or chronic nephritis; nor are they likely to be resolved in the foreseeable future by fortuitous changes in ways of life such as those that initiated the decline of the infections. (This is not to say that postnatal diseases are not attributable mainly to recent changes in ways of life.) What is in question is not the value of medical research, but the kinds of research that are likely to be successful with different classes of disease problems.

Historians recognize that scientific progress has often been retarded by psychological blocks, by inadequate conceptualization of problems for whose solution the evidence was already available. The delay for more than 1000 years in applying knowledge of optics to the study of the eye is a remarkable example. The dominance of a mechanistic approach to the problems of disease since the seventeenth century has caused us to overlook the enormous contribution from modification of disease origins in the past, and to underestimate its potential for the future. If we had been thinking of disease origins as well as mechanisms, would it have taken quite so long to suspect the importance of smoking, refinement of food and lack of exercise in respiratory, intestinal and cardiovascular disease?

There is no simple basis on which to decide the balance between preventive and therapeutic measures. It is a problem that confronts society in many fields, and reformers, if they are to be trusted, need to feel for the present and think for the future. We cannot respect the judgement of people who are so preoccupied with the present that they give no thought to what is to follow; but we cannot trust the motives of those who can ignore existing problems when designing a future blueprint.

Index